Superfoods

FOR
DUMMIES®

PORTABLE EDITION

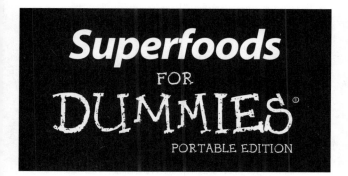

Superfoods FOR DUMMIES®
PORTABLE EDITION

by Brent Agin, MD,
and Shereen Jegtvig, MS

WILEY

Wiley Publishing, Inc.

Superfoods For Dummies,® Portable Edition

Published by
Wiley Publishing, Inc.
111 River St.
Hoboken, NJ 07030-5774
www.wiley.com

For general information on our other products and services, please contact our Customer Care Department within the U.S. at 877-762-2974, outside the U.S. at 317-572-3993, or fax 317-572-4002.

For technical support, please visit www.wiley.com/techsupport.

Wiley also publishes its books in a variety of electronic formats. Some content that appears in print may not be available in electronic books.

ISBN: 978-0-470-59192-5

Manufactured in the United States of America

10 9 8 7 6 5 4 3 2 1

Publisher's Acknowledgements

Editor: Corbin Collins
Composition Services: Indianapolis Composition Services Department
Cover photo: © Ichiro

WILEY

Table of Contents

Introduction

. . . .

*T*he power of food to help or hurt you is quite amazing. We've both seen the health of patients improve dramatically when they break their junk-food habits and turn to healthful foods instead. And we know that when patients understand the importance of nutrition, they're more likely to support a healthful diet.

Superfoods give you the most bang for your dietary buck. We think these foods are extra-special because they can improve health and prevent disease, and we have the science to back up these claims. Most superfoods are easy to find, but we also introduce you to some lesser-known superfoods.

What's in it for you? Maybe you want to be more energetic, lose weight, reduce your cholesterol, or lower your blood pressure. No matter what your reason for being interested in superfoods, we know that once you feel the benefits, you'll want to keep these superfoods in your diet for a lifetime.

About This Book

If we tried to write down everything there is to know about food, nutrition, diet, and health in this one book, you'd have to add a new room onto your home just to store it because such a book would be enormous. So, in the interest of practicality, we give you a quick overview of nutrition, then jump right into the superfoods. We do much more than just give you a list of healthful foods, though. Along the way we explain how you can benefit from adding superfoods to your diet and give you tips and how-to's for buying your superfoods. Then we tell you how to prepare them so they'll continue to be super and how to serve them so they'll be absolutely delicious. Here are a few of the points we explore:

- ✔ **Why you and your family need superfoods:** The rationale for eating them

- ✔ **What makes superfoods so super:** The science behind the food

- ✔ **Where you can find superfoods:** Grocery stores, specialty shops, and online sources

- ✔ **How to prepare and enjoy superfoods:** Cooking instructions and easy superfood recipes

Every chapter in this book is written to stand on its own, and we've included lots of examples and tips so you can start eating more superfoods right away.

Conventions Used in This Book

We use the following conventions throughout the text to make things consistent and easy to understand:

- ✔ New words or terms are in *italics,* closely followed by an easy-to-understand definition.

- ✔ **Bold** is highlights the action parts of numbered steps and key words in bulleted lists.

- ✔ When we discuss scientific research, we give you the source of that research; titles of medical and scientific journals are in *italics.*

Foolish Assumptions

This book is for anyone interested in exploring foods that not only taste great but have the potential to make you feel better and live longer. In writing this book, we assume that you, the reader, fall into one or more of the following categories:

- ✔ You're a parent looking for some guidance on nutrition and the right foods to create a balanced diet for healthy kids.

- ✔ You're a personal trainer, health instructor, or someone otherwise involved in healthy living, and you want to expand your knowledge of how you can help your clients improve their diets.

- ✔ You have medical conditions that may improve by eating superfoods.

- ✔ You're over your ideal weight and want to know how eating superfoods can help you lose weight.

- ✔ You're underweight and you're searching for healthful ways to add calories without eating junk foods.

- ✔ You already eat right, but you're looking for new foods that can add more vitamins, minerals, and antioxidants to your diet.

- ✔ You're a chef or a restaurant owner who wants easy ways to add superfoods to your recipes to make your dishes even healthier.

- ✔ You're willing to make dietary changes and stick with them until eating healthful foods is a habit.

Icons Used in This Book

This book uses *icons* — small graphics in the margins — to help you quickly recognize especially important information in the text. Here are the icons we use and what they mean:

This icon appears whenever an idea or item can save you time, money, or stress as you add superfoods to your diet. These include cooking and shopping tips, plus ideas for incorporating superfoods into some of your favorite dishes.

 Any time you see this icon, you know the information that follows is so important that it's worth reading more than once.

 This icon flags information that highlights dangers to your health or well-being.

 This icon points out recipes that are vegetarian.

Where to Go from Here

The *For Dummies* books are organized in such a way that you can surf through any of the chapters and find useful information without having to start at Chapter 1. We (naturally) encourage you to read the whole book, but this structure makes it very easy to start with the topics that interest you the most.

If you already know a lot about superfoods, turn to Chapters 6 and 7 for some great superfood recipes. If you're curious about what superfoods can do for your overall health and sense of well-being, start with Chapter 2. Or read all the chapters in order . . . you rebel.

If you want even more advice on superfoods, check out the full-size version of *Superfoods For Dummies*. Simply head to your local book seller or go to www. dummies.com!

Chapter 1

Appreciating the Ageless Wonders of Superfoods

- -

In This Chapter

▶ Discovering the healthy benefits of superfoods

▶ Unlocking anti-aging abilities

- -

*P*eople today typically eat for pleasure rather than for good nutrition. Unfortunately, there just aren't many health benefits in most of the foods we eat for pleasure. If eating a candy bar could decrease your blood pressure or reduce your risk for cancer, we'd have one heck of a healthy population — but this just isn't the case.

One of the reasons people don't choose healthier food is because they haven't been educated on the actual health benefits of eating the good stuff. But read on, because in this chapter you find out how the foods you eat can affect — and even improve — your health.

Boosting Your Immune System

As you may expect, superfoods are good immune system boosters, helping your body fight and prevent various diseases. Research on certain foods' abilities to strengthen immune function, fight against heart disease, prevent cancer, and lower the risk of other inflammatory diseases has been piling up. Of course, cancer is much less common than colds and minor infections. Fortunately, superfoods can help with everyday ailments, too. Here are two good examples:

- ✔ **Resveratrol,** a compound found in red wine, has antiviral properties and can help prevent common cold viruses from taking hold in your body.

- ✔ **Garlic** has been used as a natural antibiotic for more than a century. Louis Pasteur studied the use of garlic as an antibiotic and found that it killed bacteria in the lab.

 If you're on any medications, see your doctor before you add high doses of garlic to your regimen. Garlic can interfere with certain medication functions.

Helping Your Heart

Your heart pumps about 2,000 gallons of blood throughout your body every day, but most people don't appreciate what a workload that is. Unfortunately, sometimes it takes a serious medical condition to become aware of your heart — by which time you may already have heart disease.

Heart disease is the leading cause of death in men and women, so reducing risks should be a priority for both genders. Superfoods can help by tackling *cholesterol* (a fat-like substance that helps produce cell membranes and hormones) and *triglycerides* (a type of fat that makes up a portion of the cholesterol), believed to be major risk factors for cardiovascular disease.

Superfoods work to keep your heart healthy and improve your ticker's longevity without the potential side effects or expense of cholesterol-lowering prescription medications. They can really make a difference in your heart's health. Here's how:

- ✔ Eating superfoods means you're improving your overall diet and getting the vitamins and minerals you need every day — without extra calories. Too many extra calories cause elevations in triglycerides and an increased risk for heart disease.

- ✔ Some superfoods, such as colorful fruits and vegetables, contain natural disease-fighting substances called *flavonoids*. These can reduce inflammation of your arteries, decrease your cholesterol, lower your blood pressure, and stimulate antioxidant activity.

- ✔ Fish, nuts, and seeds contain healthful polyunsaturated fatty acids that keep your cholesterol in check. Fish oil (omega-3 fatty acids) is particularly super because it also helps regulate your heartbeat and blood pressure.

- ✔ Fruits, vegetables, and oatmeal all contain dietary fiber that lowers cholesterol and helps keep you feeling full, which can prevent overeating, a risk factor for heart disease.

Losing Weight

More than 70 percent of the adult population in the United States is overweight, and a third of that population is obese. *Overweight* is defined as having a *body mass index* (BMI) over 25. Adults with a BMI over 30 are considered *obese*. Obesity is the second most preventable health risk, just behind smoking. It's a problem worldwide but more so in the United States — and it just keeps getting bigger.

As with heart disease, poor eating habits and physical inactivity are largely responsible for weight gain. Weight loss isn't easy, but for many people it's necessary to restore and maintain good health. Eating superfoods can help you lose weight.

Protecting Against Cancer

Cancer is the second leading cause of death in the United States, just behind heart disease. Although many people believe that cancer is an uncontrollable health condition, evidence suggests otherwise. Some superfoods may help prevent cancer and improve the well-being of cancer patients.

 Many superfoods have cancer-fighting proper-ties. In general, you should seek those foods with the highest amounts of phytochemicals, fiber, and antioxidants. For example:

- ✔ Lycopene, a phytochemical found in tomatoes, may reduce the risk of prostate cancer and other cancers, according to the American Cancer Society.

- ✔ Berries contain phytochemicals that have been shown to help fight the development of cancer. These phytochemicals trigger antioxidant reac-tions that neutralize damage to your cells.

- ✔ Red wine contains two polyphenols called cate-chins and resveratrol, both of which provide cancer protection by inhibiting the growth of cancer cells.

- ✔ Broccoli contains a chemical that has been found to slow the progression of cancer cells, especially hormone-sensitive cancers such as breast and ovarian cancer.

- ✔ Several studies support the theory that garlic and garlic extracts can reduce the risk of cancer.

- ✔ Several beans (legumes) are great sources of fiber, which has been proved to help reduce inflammation in the colon and has been associated with a reduction of colon cancer.

Improving Digestion

Most people suffer digestive stress at one time or another. For example, constipation is common and can lead to abdominal bloating, hemorrhoids, and unnecessary pain. Indigestion or acid reflux (heartburn) is a common cause of emergency department visits and can lead to damage in the esophagus if not treated. Regularity of the digestive system is important for the proper metabolism of the foods you eat so they can be used by the body.

One way to help your digestive system is to eat foods with lots of fiber. The average diet consists of about 10 grams of fiber a day — far less than the 25 to 40 grams per day that your body needs. Boost your fiber intake by adding superfood fruits, vegetables, nuts, grains, and legumes, such as the following, to your diet:

- ✔ Almonds
- ✔ Apples
- ✔ Avocados
- ✔ Black beans
- ✔ Blueberries
- ✔ Broccoli
- ✔ Chia
- ✔ Lentils

✔ Lima beans

✔ Oatmeal

✔ Quinoa

✔ Soy beans

 Water isn't on our list of superfoods, but it's a great addition to your diet to help some of the super-fiber foods work better. Drinking half your body weight (in ounces!) of water each day helps counter the fluids that fiber absorbs — if you weigh 120 pounds, for example, you should aim to drink 60 ounces of water a day.

A fiber primer

If you aren't sure what fiber is and why it's good for you, you're not alone. *Fiber* is the part of plant foods (fruits, vegetables, grains) that can't be broken down by your digestive system. Fiber is important for your health — it keeps your digestive system healthy and helps to control blood sugar levels.

There are two types of fiber:

✔ **Insoluble fiber:** This type of fiber doesn't dissolve in water and cannot be digested. It absorbs water and bulks the stool to help regulate bowel movements. Insoluble fiber is found in grains and some vegetables.

✔ **Soluble fiber:** This type of fiber dissolves in water, forming a gel-like substance that moves through the intestines. Found in fruits, vegetables, and legumes, soluble fiber is associated with lowering cholesterol and controlling blood sugar.

A food is considered to have a high fiber content when it has more than five grams of fiber per serving.

Easing Inflammation

When it comes to staying healthy, your body is always in a tug-of-war with detriments like pollution, unhealthy foods, smoke, too much alcohol, excessive sunlight, and even the side effects of fighting infections and digesting high-fat meals. Exposure to these things causes cell damage and *inflammation* (the body's response to this damage, such as tissue swelling, redness, and triggering of the immune system). *Chronic inflammation,* or inflammation that happens over and over again, can lead to problems in the joints, heart, colon, and even skin.

Your body works hard to fight inflammation and cell damage. You can give your body an edge by eating superfoods rich in antioxidants and prostaglandins, which we discuss in the following sections.

The role of antioxidants

Antioxidants are natural substances, such as the compounds that give fruits and vegetables their colors, and vitamins like C and E, which fight cell damage. They work to fight inflammation by neutralizing free radicals in the body. *Free radicals* are unstable molecules that can travel throughout the body trying to take particles from healthy cells — a process that creates more free radicals. Free radicals damage cells, causing inflammation and starting a chain reaction in tissues as more and more cells become affected.

Superfoods are packed with antioxidants that move through the body and stop the free radicals so they don't damage healthy cells. Blueberries, broccoli, cranberries, green tea, pomegranates, and spinach are some superfoods that have the most powerful antioxidant properties.

Fats and inflammation

Your body makes chemicals called *prostaglandins* that contribute to starting or stopping inflammation reactions in your body (depending on the type of prostaglandins). Have you ever taken aspirin or ibuprofen for a headache? These medicines stop inflammation by blocking the prostaglandins.

Some foods can increase the amount of inflammatory prostaglandins (the bad ones) and decrease the amount of anti-inflammatory prostaglandins (the good ones) in your body. Eating these foods increases inflammation in your body. Eating a diet high in *saturated fat* (a type of fat found in red meat) is a major cause of this prostaglandin imbalance and the resulting inflammation. Fortunately, superfoods combat that inflammation.

Unlike saturated fats, unsaturated fats are good for the body. They come in two forms: polyunsaturated and monounsaturated.

A type of polyunsaturated fat known as omega-3 fatty acids is especially good for you. Omega-3s have been found to reduce inflammation. Eating foods rich in omega-3 can help prevent heart disease, cancer, and arthritis.

You have to get these fats from the foods you eat; your body can't produce them. So if you don't get enough from your diet, it's important to take a quality supplement.

Monounsaturated fat is also good for you. It's the fat found in olive oil, and it may be one reason why people who eat Mediterranean diets tend to be very healthy.

The following superfoods are packed with good poly- and monounsaturated fats and can help pump up your body's anti-inflammatory defense system:

✔ Fish and seafood contain lots of omega-3 fats.

✔ Chia, walnuts, and flax seeds are great plant sources of omega-3s.

✔ Avocados and olive oil are healthy monounsaturated fats.

Aging Beautifully

Superfoods do a lot of things, but trying to turn a frog into a prince may be pushing it. Offering some benefits that can help you live a longer and more vigorous life, however, is definitely within their call of duty.

 Eating superfoods helps you stay youthful, and the earlier you start with superfoods, the more age-defying benefits you can gain.

Keeping that youthful glow

The health and beauty sections of drugstores are stuffed with creams, lotions, cleansers, moisturizers, and makeup designed to minimize the signs of aging. But a diet that includes superfoods can do just as much — and even more — to keep your skin healthy and young-looking.

The skin deals with so many different factors — sun, pollution, extreme weather, and other irritants — that it needs a continual supply of antioxidants to help protect it. Fortunately, superfoods are chock-full of many of the main nutrients your skin needs, including:

✔ **Vitamins A, E, and C:** These help protect the skin and are vital in repairing damaged skin. Common foods that contain high levels of these vitamins include carrots (vitamin A); nuts and seeds (vitamin E); spinach (vitamins A and E); and broccoli, strawberries, and oranges (vitamin C).

✔ **Zinc and selenium:** Zinc is active in the synthesis of collagen. Pumpkin seeds are an excellent source of zinc, as are nuts and beans. Selenium exhibits antioxidant effects that have been found to reduce skin cancer. Selenium is found in fish and nuts.

✔ **Bioflavonoids:** *Bioflavonoids* are the pigments found in the skins of colorful fruits and vegetables. These pigments contain concentrated antioxidants that are more powerful than vitamins. They help increase vitamin C levels and reduce destruction of collagen in the skin.

✔ **Alpha-lipoic acid (ALA):** This is a fatty acid made by the body and found in foods such as broccoli and spinach. Although the body produces ALA, it doesn't make nearly enough to be helpful for fighting disease and inflammation.

Pumping up your pep

When you feel a drop in your energy level or you've hit a midday slump, skip the coffee, chocolate, or "energy" drink, which may contain artificial stimulants and are usually high in sugar. Instead, go natural and use superfoods to put some pep in your step.

Getting a natural boost of energy is important not only for getting through your daily routine, but also for summoning extra energy to tackle your exercise program or other activities. When you use the right foods and eat small meals throughout the day, you can ramp up your metabolism and get that extra energy you need.

If you're on the go and can't find the time to grab a healthy meal, these superfoods can be a great option:

✔ **Goji berries:** Rich in antioxidants, goji berries help boost energy and enhance your mood.

✔ **Green tea:** The *American Journal of Clinical Nutrition* found that green tea's effect on energy was similar to that of caffeine.

✔ **Chia seed:** Chia seeds can absorb ten times their weight and are slow to digest, offering sustained energy for several hours. You can add chia seeds to protein shakes or other meals to get sustained energy throughout the day.

✔ **Quinoa:** This protein-rich seed, though considered a grain, is actually a leafy plant that's related to spinach and beets, and it can give you a power punch.

Seeing and believing

Many bodily functions change with age, and vision is no exception. Many people develop the need for some type of visual correction as they grow older. Just like other age-related conditions that can be alleviated by superfoods, the eyes can be aided by the following superfood constituents:

✔ **Beta carotene:** You've probably heard that eating carrots is supposed to help improve your vision and reduce your risk for *macular degeneration,* a progressive disease of the retina that affects the light-sensing cells, causing blurring or blind spots in your central vision. That's because carrots contain a lot of beta carotene, a precursor to vitamin A. Beta carotene is virtually a staple ingredient in vision-related nutritional supplements.

✔ **Acanthocyanins:** These are bioflavonoids that give color to the skin of fruits and veggies. Their antioxidant properties help protect not only your eyes, but other organ systems as well.

✔ **Lutein:** Lutein is concentrated in your retinas. Carrots have high levels of lutein. Other good sources are broccoli, spinach, kale, and orange and yellow fruits.

✔ **Omega-3 fatty acids:** Omega-3s protect the light-sensing cells in your eyes. Eating fish and other foods that contain omega-3s can reduce the risk of developing macular degeneration and cataracts.

Chapter 2

Bringing Superfoods into Your Life

- -

In This Chapter

▶ Getting superfoods into your diet

▶ Figuring out how much to eat

▶ Finding superfoods in restaurants

- -

Choosing superfoods is beneficial no matter what the rest of your diet is like, but the results are magnified when those superfoods are incorporated into a diet that's healthful overall.

Getting started isn't all that difficult, and after you get moving, you'll want to keep your superfoods diet going, even at restaurants and parties. In this chapter, you discover how to incorporate superfoods into your lifestyle — at home, at work, or at play.

Transforming Your Diet into a Superfoods Diet

A superfoods diet isn't like a fad diet or crash diet that requires you to give up or severely restrict any nutrients. A healthy diet includes foods of all kinds, because when you eliminate certain food groups or nutrients (such as bread and cereals, carbohydrates, or fats), you feel deprived, and then you go off whatever diet you were on. By choosing a superfoods diet, you reduce the amounts of not-so-healthy foods you eat and focus on adding lots of healthy (and delicious) foods from all the food groups.

The changes you make in your diet will last your whole life. You do need to sacrifice a little bit, like cutting way back on eating greasy processed foods and sugary snacks, but the payback is enjoying a healthy, youthful body.

Making the shift: Foods you should eat more or less of

Start with a basic healthy diet. Eat less of the foods that are bad for you and more of the foods that are good for you. First, restrict these foods:

- ✔ **Extra added sugar, including sucrose and high fructose corn syrup:** Replace regular soda with caffeine-free diet soda or water. Cut back on candy, pastries, and other sweets. Sweeteners add calories fast but don't add any nutrition. Instead, eat superfood fruits that are naturally sweet, and you won't miss the sugar.

- ✔ **Saturated and trans fats:** Cut back on fatty red meats, switch to nonfat milk, and avoid processed foods and stick margarines that have "partially hydrogenated oil" as an ingredient. Choose seafood, skinless chicken, turkey, lean beef, and pork, but avoid anything that's deep-fried. Substitute superfood fish and legumes for red meats to get the protein you need without the saturated fats. Replace trans fat–laden stick margarine with olive oil or with margarines made with olive oil, flax oil, or canola oil.

✔ **Extra sodium:** It's okay to sprinkle some salt on your foods, but watch out for extra salt and sodium hidden in highly processed and canned foods and most boxed meal mixes. Superfoods in their natural forms are low in sodium. Look for low-sodium versions of canned foods, or opt for fresh or frozen whenever possible.

 Replace the restricted items in the preceding list with healthier alternatives by eating more of these:

✔ **Healthy fats:** Eat foods rich in omega-3 fatty acids, such as fish, flax, chia, pumpkin seeds, and canola oil. Choose olive oil, avocado, and nuts for healthy polyunsaturated and monounsaturated fats.

✔ **Fiber:** Increase your intake of fruits, vegetables, and whole grains. Most days you should choose more vegetables than fruits. And consume whole-grain breads, cereals, and pasta to add much-needed fiber.

✔ **Healthy proteins:** The best protein sources include meats, seafood, eggs, dairy products, nuts, and legumes. What makes a protein source healthful is not the type of protein, but how that source is prepared. For example, grilled shrimp is good, but shrimp scampi is high in saturated fat and bad for your heart and arteries.

Fitting in superfoods every day

To start your superfoods diet, eat at least two superfoods each day. Eat one at breakfast or as a snack, and eat another at lunch or dinner. When this becomes a habit, add a third superfood, and eventually a fourth.

As you get used to choosing nutritious foods for every meal, many of your choices will automatically be superfoods.

Looking at your dietary needs for a typical day, you can see how easily superfoods can fit in. The United States Department of Agriculture (USDA) has designed a food pyramid to help you figure out how many foods you need to eat from each food group every day. Here's what the food pyramid calls for:

- **Six to eleven servings from the bread and cereal group:** At least half of these servings should be whole grains. Superfood grains — oats and quinoa — fit in nicely here. Other good choices include 100 percent whole wheat, popcorn, cornmeal, brown rice, and barley.

- **Five to nine servings of fruits and vegetables:** All fruits and vegetables are good for you. It's best to choose a few more vegetables than fruits. Superfood fruits and vegetables are even better because they're rich in nutrients and fiber.

- **Three servings of dairy or calcium-fortified foods:** Yogurt is really quite good for you because it contains *probiotics* (friendly bacteria that keep your gut healthy). Yogurt works with superfoods, too, because you can add fruit and nuts.

- **Two to three servings of meat and dry beans:** The best meats for this category are low-fat meats, so lean beef, pork, eggs, skinless chicken, turkey, fish, and seafood are good choices. Superfoods for this group include salmon, tuna, sardines, trout, and legumes.

- **Fats and oils:** You get the fats you need from the foods you eat, including fish, meats, nuts, seeds, dressings, and any cooking oil you use. Fish does double duty as a superfood protein source and a healthful fat. Other good fats come from a variety of superfoods, including flax, pumpkin seeds, olive oil, avocado, and chia.

✔ **Discretionary calories:** This is where your treats — sodas, cookies, cakes, and candy — fit in, and the allotment is only about 100 to 200 calories per day. It's not much, but a little bit of these treats can keep cravings at bay. Choose your superfood treats wisely. For example, enjoy 1 ounce of dark chocolate or one 5-ounce glass of wine.

 Pump up the amount of fruits and vegetables you eat because this is the easiest way to add more superfoods, given that many fruits and vegetables are superfoods.

Portion control: Knowing serving sizes

Understanding serving sizes is crucial for controlling portion sizes and getting enough (or avoiding getting too much) of certain foods.

 A serving and a portion are not necessarily the same. A *serving* is a measured amount, such as an 8-ounce glass of milk or ½ cup of sliced fruit. A *portion* is the amount of food that you choose to eat. So while that giant bagel you buy at the coffee shop is only one *portion,* it may really be equal to four or five *servings* from the bread and cereal group. The following list identifies what constitutes a serving of some common foods:

✔ **Fruits:** One serving of fruit is equal to ½ cup of sliced fruit or half of a large whole fruit. Half a cup is about the size of half a baseball.

✔ **Vegetables:** One serving of vegetables is also ½ cup. Because *green leafy* vegetables are so low in calories, one serving is about 1 to 2 cups.

✔ **Breads and cereals:** One slice of bread counts as a serving in the cereal group. A serving of rice or pasta equals ½ cup.

✔ **Fats and oils:** One serving of oil or fat is 1 teaspoon, which is about the size of the tip of your thumb. Many fats are found in your protein sources, like nuts. One serving of nuts is 1 ounce, or about 25 almonds or 9 walnuts.

✔ **Proteins:** One serving of protein is equal to 3 ounces of meat, fish, or poultry, which is about the size of a deck of cards. A serving of a thinner fillet of fish is about the size of a checkbook. One egg is equal to one protein serving, and one serving of legumes is ½ cup.

When you're eating packaged foods, you can figure out how much of it constitutes one serving by looking at the Nutrition Facts label on the package. The USDA requires nutrition facts labeling on all packaged foods, based on servings per package.

Getting the right number of servings is important for getting enough nutrition without getting too many (or too few) calories. Most superfoods are low in calories, which allows for more servings rather than fewer. However, you still need to be careful with some superfoods, such as the nuts and oils that rack up the calories quickly if you eat too much.

Volumes of veggies

Let's start with the foods you can eat a lot of — those delicious vegetables. All of our superfood vegetables are low in calories because they're high in fiber. For example, one medium tomato has only about 25 calories, but it's packed with nutrients such as vitamin C and lutein (a powerful antioxidant). Green and other colorful vegetables are also low in calories, while being high in fiber and nutrients.

Eat several servings of vegetables every day. The USDA food pyramid suggests 2 cups at a minimum (at least three servings), but, for good health, you can eat much more than that — up to 4 cups each day.

Scores of fruits

You can also eat many servings of fruit as long as they're whole fruits or used as ingredients in healthy recipes. An apple is good for you; a piece of apple pie isn't. Fruit generally has more calories than vegetables, so keep that in mind if you're watching calories. An orange or an apple has about 80 calories — more than a tomato, but way less than a candy bar.

The USDA food pyramid includes about 1½ to 2 cups of fruit in a balanced diet (three to four of your daily five to nine servings of fruits and vegetables). That's about the same as eating one apple and half a banana. But because fruits are so good for you, feel free to eat 2½ to 3 cups every day.

Being smart with fish

Our superfood fish is rich in omega-3 fatty acids, and the American Heart Association recommends that you should eat fish at least twice a week. There are valid concerns about mercury toxicity in fish, so it may be smart to limit your weekly intake to about 12 ounces, or three to four servings.

Picking fats prudently

Nuts such as almonds and walnuts are so delicious that it's easy to get carried away when you eat them. Although the fats they contain are healthful fats, they also contain calories that need to be counted if you're watching your weight. If you want to lose weight, limit your servings of nuts and seeds to just one per day (about 25 almonds or 9 walnuts). If you need to gain weight, eating extra servings of nuts is a good way to get extra nutritious calories.

Olive oil is another superfood because the fats it contains are good for your heart. But olive oil is also high in calories. It's important to balance the healthful properties of good fats with the extra calories that can lead to weight gain, so measure olive oil carefully when you use it.

Adding Superfoods to Your Meals

Another important step in getting started with a superfoods diet is getting those superfoods into your meals. Some of your favorite recipes may already have superfoods as ingredients.

If you use recipes that don't call for superfoods, look for ways to incorporate them. You may be able to substitute superfoods for some ingredients (like olive oil for vegetable oil), or simply add a superfood to a dish (sprinkle chopped almonds on your veggie side dish).

Make superfoods a part of every meal: breakfast, lunch, and dinner. In the next three sections, we show you how.

Starting your day with superfoods

Breakfast is a good time to get some superfoods into your stomach.

If you're used to eating sweet stuff in the morning, reduce the sugar and get your sweetness fix from superfood fruits. Instead of sugar-frosted breakfast flakes, eat a bowl of whole-grain cereal topped with berries or banana slices. (If you choose oatmeal to go with those berries, you already have two superfoods.)

You can make your omelets into superfood omelets when you cut back on the cheese and meats and add vegetables like tomatoes, spinach, or broccoli.

Need your morning caffeine fix? Switch out your coffee for green tea, which has antioxidants that may prevent cancer and still has a little caffeine to perk you up.

If you usually skip breakfast, use the superfoods to get you into the healthy habit of eating something before work or school. Grab a banana and a handful of pecans, and you're ready to head out the door.

Packing healthier lunches and snacks

When you're packing your lunch, sandwiches can be made with whole-grain bread, and you can add an extra slice of tomato or use spinach leaves in place of lettuce. Pack crunchy vegetables instead of chips.

When you don't want a sandwich, you can pack vegetable soup. If you have a refrigerator and microwave at work, you can bring leftover salmon from dinner the night before. You can also pack a salad, made of superfood vegetables, fruits, and nuts, in a plastic container. Pour your salad dressing into a separate container or zip-top bag so your salad isn't soggy by lunchtime.

Round out your superfoods lunch with a healthy beverage like 100 percent fruit or vegetable juice instead of soda.

Superfood supplements

Superfood supplements are really exploding onto the scene, and many manufacturers claim they can get more of some of the superfood qualities in supplements than you can get by eating healthful foods. Superfood supplements give your nutrition a boost by concentrating some of the nutrients, but they can't replace the healthy foods in your diet. You need to continue to eat wholesome foods that provide you with fiber, protein, and other nutrients that build your body and keep you strong. Eating a junk food diet is unhealthy no matter what supplements you take.

Superfood supplements are great for those times when you're under a lot of stress, trying to lose weight, or fighting infections, or if you're a picky eater. But your best option still is to get the energy-building properties you need from the food you eat, rather than solely from a supplement bottle.

Keep healthy snacks at work so you won't be tempted to raid the vending machines. Dried fruits and nuts keep well and are portable, so you can take them wherever you go.

Serving super dinner dishes

There are several ways to get superfoods into your dinners. Consider these options:

- ✔ Start your dinner with a garden salad made with superfood vegetables on spinach leaves and topped with a few chopped nuts. You can even serve a big salad as a meal in itself.

- ✔ Choose superfoods as side dishes; they can be as simple as steamed broccoli with a little lemon, or a bit fancier. Make your side dishes colorful — the color in vegetables indicates anti-oxidant protection.

✔ Serve superfood fish as a main dish. Salmon is particularly good because of its high omega-3 fatty acid content. Tuna is good, and so is trout.

✔ End your meal with superfoods such as berries and cream for a delicious and nutritious dessert.

Eating Out with Superfoods

Americans spend about half of their food dollars in restaurants. It's easy to go to a restaurant, but it's important to remember two things: Many menu selections are high in calories, and they're served in huge portions.

Frequently dining out probably isn't the best way to maintain a healthy diet. But if you do eat many of your meals out, you can make better menu choices and even find a few superfoods in restaurants.

Finding fast-food superfood

Our best advice is to avoid fast-food places when you can. When you do need to eat fast food, choose small portions and look for superfoods.

The best fast-food restaurants are the sub sandwich shops. There, you can choose lean meats, including tuna, and add tomatoes along with other vegetables. Opt for just a little dressing — sub shops usually don't use healthy oils.

 Here are some tips for finding superfoods at fast-food restaurants:

✔ Choose a side salad or fruit, like apple slices, instead of greasy fries.

✔ Order apple or orange juice instead of soda.

✔ Eat a meal-sized salad for lunch. Look for salads with grilled, low-fat meats, or just fruits and vegetables.

Ordering superfoods at sit-down restaurants

Sit-down restaurants usually have more menu choices than fast-food restaurants. The key to eating a superfoods diet in a sit-down restaurant is to choose wisely and not be tempted by the unhealthy foods.

Here are some tips for finding superfoods at sit-down restaurants:

✔ Look for superfoods in the salads.

✔ Ask what the vegetable of the day is when one is offered.

✔ Check out the soup of the day.

✔ Order fish that has been baked or broiled.

✔ Look for vegetarian meals, which often include some superfoods.

✔ Ask for fruit for dessert.

Chapter 3

Singling Out Super-Duper Superfoods

*T*his chapter gives you the best of the best superfoods. These foods pack the highest nutritional punch and can make the biggest impact on your health. We chose these foods based on nutritional content, versatility, availability, and ease of storage.

Seeing What Salmon Has to Offer

Salmon is a very richly flavored fish found in cold ocean waters. It's a source of several vitamins and minerals and has plenty of protein. It also has the highest levels of omega-3 fatty acids of commercially available fish.

Getting the lowdown on nutrition

Salmon is a good source of healthful protein, vitamins, and minerals. A 6-ounce salmon fillet has 240 calories and favorable amounts of these important nutrients:

- ✔ **Magnesium** helps regulate muscle contractions and can also help relax the muscles within artery walls. This makes magnesium important in reducing migraines and blood pressure.

- ✔ **Potassium** helps the heart beat regularly and it supports the nervous system.

- ✔ **Selenium** binds with protein to become an antioxidant and can help reduce the risk of cancer.

- ✔ **B vitamins** consist of eight individual vitamins that are important for your immune system, metabolism, and cognition.

- ✔ **Omega-3 fats** help reduce inflammation in muscles and the inflammation associated with heart disease. Omega-3 fats reduce levels of bad cholesterol and can help lower blood pressure.

Serving up salmon

Buying and preparing salmon is a cinch. Fresh salmon may be available at your local grocery store (look for fillets that are pinkish in color with shiny skin and firm flesh), or you may find frozen salmon fillets, smoked salmon, or canned salmon chunks — they're all good for you. Salmon is also commonly found on the menus of many restaurants. Salmon could be the healthiest choice on the menu because it's usually baked, grilled, or broiled and served with vegetables and salad.

Salmon's fat content makes it easy to cook because it's less likely to become dry if you overcook it. Salmon also cooks quickly. Broil it about 10 minutes per each inch of thickness, or bake fillets at 350 degrees Fahrenheit for about 20 minutes.

Canned salmon is convenient and ready to use for sandwiches, salads, and recipes like salmon cakes.

Getting Strong with Spinach

Spinach is a leafy green vegetable rich in nutrients, including many important vitamins and minerals, plus fiber. Eat spinach raw or cooked. Either way it's low in calories — 1 cup of raw spinach has just 7 calories, while a cup of cooked spinach has about 32 calories (cooked spinach is denser). Because spinach is so nutritious, we suggest you eat it four times per week.

Bursting with antioxidant protection

Spinach is a good source of vitamins A, E, and K. All the cells in your body need vitamin A to promote reproduction through cell division. Vitamin E may help to prevent some cancers and cardiovascular disease, and vitamin K helps your blood to clot properly. Spinach also provides large amounts of beta carotene, which functions as an antioxidant that protects your body's cells.

Spinach is rich in folate, potassium, and magnesium, which are important for your cardiovascular system and for healthy nerves and muscles. Spinach is also a good plant source of iron (perfect for vegetarians).

When you eat spinach, you reap a host of health benefits, including the following:

✔ **Keeping cancer at bay:** The journal *Nutrition and Cancer* reported in 2003 that several antioxidant compounds in spinach have anti-inflammatory and anti-cancer properties. A 2004 article in *The Journal of the National Cancer Institute* stated that folate may reduce the risk of ovarian cancer.

✔ **Maintaining heart health:** The folate in spinach reduces homocysteine levels that are associated with an elevated risk of cardiovascular disease. The antioxidant lutein has been shown to reduce inflammation and plaque build-up in the arteries. Spinach also improves heart health with an ample amount of potassium while being naturally low in sodium.

If you have high blood pressure, be sure to choose fresh or frozen spinach to avoid sodium. If you want canned spinach, look for a brand that's low in sodium.

✔ **Strengthening bones:** Vitamin K activates the protein osteocalcin that's involved in bone formation. A vitamin K deficiency may lead to weaker bones. Spinach also contains magnesium and calcium, which are also helpful for strong bones. However, the calcium in spinach is not absorbed as easily as calcium in dairy products, due to a substance called *oxalic acid* that's also in spinach.

✔ **Seeing clearly:** Your eyes need vitamin A to function properly because one form of vitamin A, retinal, is an important component of your retina. Lutein, vitamin E, and beta carotene have all been studied for their ability to impair the development of macular degeneration, the leading cause of blindness in the elderly.

✔ **Staying sharp:** The antioxidants found in spinach help to keep your mind sharp. *The Annals of the New York Academy of Sciences* reported in 2007 that diets rich in fruits and vegetables, especially berries and spinach, help to maximize cognitive function long into old age. According to the journal *Clinical Nutrition* in 2008, decreased blood levels of B vitamins, including folate, correlate with a decline in cognitive function.

While folate appears to be important for healthy brain function, folic acid supplements may not do the trick. A 2008 study in *The Journal of the American Medical Association* reported that B vitamin supplementation had no positive effect on slowing the progression of Alzheimer's disease. For optimal brain function, rely on fruits and vegetables rather than folic acid supplements.

✔ **Boosting energy:** Spinach contains iron and folate, both of which are important for preventing anemia. This can be especially important for women who regularly have heavy menstrual periods.

✔ **Preventing spinal cord malformation:** Women who are deficient in folate are much more likely to give birth to babies with spina bifida, which affects the spinal cord and bones.

✔ **Fighting infections:** Vitamin A acts as an immune system regulator by making white blood cells that kill viruses and bacteria. Vitamin E, which is found in spinach, also impacts immune function. *The Journal of the American Medical Association* published a study in 2004 showing that extra vitamin E improved the immune systems of the elderly.

Selecting and savoring spinach

Fresh spinach is available year-round in just about every grocery store, usually right next to the salad greens. In fact, you can substitute spinach for lettuce in many salads to make them healthier. Choose fresh spinach that is dark green in color and looks fresh.

Frozen and canned spinach are also available. Canned spinach usually contains added sodium, so if you're on a sodium-restricted diet, be sure to read the labels to find brands with little or no sodium added.

Store unwashed spinach in your refrigerator until you want to use it — washing the leaves beforehand causes them to deteriorate. Rinse the leaves with cold water thoroughly to remove dirt and bugs.

 You can add spinach to pasta sauce or use it as a pizza topping. Fresh spinach leaves can also replace lettuce on sandwiches. Spinach can also be incorporated into mashed potato recipes or added to stuffing. Make breakfast healthier by using spinach in your omelets and quiches.

The Fruit that Eats Like a Vegetable: The Tomato

Tomatoes contain several vitamins, and the beautiful red coloring holds phytochemicals that support your heart, immune system, and vision and may prevent cancer. One tomato gives you half the vitamin C you need for the day. Tomatoes are also a good source of fiber, which helps keep your digestive system healthy.

Loving the perks of lycopene and more

Tomatoes offer vitamins A and C, plus lutein, zeaxanthin, and lots of lycopene (a carotene that's closely related to vitamin A and beta carotene), while being very low in calories. According to an article published in 2000 in *The Canadian Medical Association Journal,* lycopene is linked to having a lower risk of cardiovascular disease and cancers.

 Lycopene is activated by heat and processing, so when you eat tomato juice, spaghetti sauce, or even ketchup, you actually get more lycopene than you would from a fresh tomato.

Tomatoes are also rich in potassium and very low in sodium, so they can be part of a healthy diet to reduce high blood pressure (just watch out for high-sodium sauces and tomato soups). We suggest that you eat tomatoes (or tomato products) five times each week to cash in on the following benefits:

- **Keeping your eyes healthy:** Vitamin A, lutein, and zeaxanthin are important for healthy vision. Research published in *The British Journal of Nutrition* in 2009 reported that those antioxidants, plus lycopene, may help to reduce the risk of retinopathy (disease of the retina inside the eye) in diabetics.

- **Protecting your heart:** In *The Canadian Medical Association Journal* in 2008, researchers stated that diets rich in tomato and tomato products reduce the risk of cardiovascular diseases, with the credit again going to lycopene. The other antioxidants in tomatoes help combat inflammation and plaque build-up in your arteries.

- **Reducing your risk of cancer:** According to the same article, eating tomatoes is associated with a reduced risk of several cancers, including prostate, breast, and digestive tract cancers. The researchers believe lycopene prevents cancer by protecting the DNA in cells.

- **Boosting your immune system (and feeling better when you have a cold):** Vitamins A and C boost your immune system, and in 2008, *The*

Journal of Nutritional Biochemistry reported that lycopene helps to reduce inflammation in your airways caused by cold viruses. Eating tomatoes may help to reduce some of your suffering when you catch a cold.

Tempting tomatoes: Selecting and serving tips

Fresh tomatoes come in a variety of shapes and sizes and are available year-round in the produce section of your grocery store, but there is a definite difference in flavor. The vine-ripened tomatoes of summer are much more flavorful than tomatoes that are harvested while immature and artificially ripened.

Choose fresh tomatoes that are a deep red in color, firm, and heavy. Avoid tomatoes with bruised skins and those that feel too squishy. Tomatoes are also sold in cans as tomato sauce, tomato pieces, or stewed whole tomatoes.

Store your fresh tomatoes, just as they are, at room temperature. Refrigerated tomatoes lose their flavor.

When you're ready to enjoy a tomato, simply rinse the skin, remove the stem, and slice or chop the tomato. Some people prefer to remove the seedy part and serve just the flesh.

Getting tomatoes into your diet is easy. Sliced tomatoes are perfect for sandwiches. Smaller pieces of tomatoes are perfect for a salad, or pop a few cherry tomatoes in your mouth as a quick snack.

Other ideas for tomatoes include topping a baked potato with home-made salsa and adding slices of sun-dried tomatoes to your favorite vegetables. Broil thick tomato slices with a little bit of parmesan cheese, garlic, and bread crumbs.

Picking Beautiful Blueberries

Blueberries burst with flavor and good health. In fact, blueberries have more antioxidants than any other commercially grown fruit. The dark blue pigment found in blueberries contains phenols called *anthocyanins* (flavonoids with powerful antioxidant capabilities). Consequently, they have many health benefits, so try to enjoy 3 or 4 cups of blueberries every week.

Tapping into the antioxidant power of blueberries

The antioxidants in blueberries protect the cells in your body from damage by free radicals. This damage can come from too much sun exposure, pollution, foods with unhealthy fats, and even as a byproduct of normal metabolism.

One cup of blueberries contains 14 milligrams of vitamin C, half a milligram of manganese (an essential trace mineral important for many chemical reactions in your body), 4 grams of fiber, and only 84 calories. Blueberries help your body in several ways:

- ✔ They keep your blood vessels strong and may lower cholesterol.

- ✔ They help prevent colon and ovarian cancer by promoting anti-cancer activity in your cells.

- ✔ They keep your vision clear by promoting healthy night vision and preventing *macular degeneration* (an age-related eye disease that's the leading cause of vision loss in the elderly).

- ✔ They keep your mind sharp and may protect you from Alzheimer's disease.

✔ They prevent urinary tract infections by preventing bacteria from sticking to the walls of your bladder.

Purchasing and preparing blueberries

Blueberries are usually easy to find in the produce and freezer sections at your grocery store. Blueberries freeze very well, and they're good for you, whether fresh or frozen.

Selecting blueberries at the grocery store is easy. Look for berries that are deep blue with little to no trace of green coloring; unlike many fruits, blueberries don't continue to ripen after they're picked. Healthy blueberries should be firm with a slight shimmer to the skin, and there should be no sign of mold.

Keep blueberries in your refrigerator. Don't wash them until you want to use them because moisture hastens deterioration. Blueberries are delicate and quite perishable, so eat them within a few days or freeze them in sturdy plastic containers.

You can easily incorporate blueberries into your superfoods diet. Traditional uses of blueberries include baked goods such as pancakes and muffins because blueberries hold up well to heat. Sprinkle some berries on your whole-grain cereal or oatmeal in the morning, or enjoy a bowl of blueberries with a little milk or cream and a few walnuts for breakfast. You can even add frozen blueberries and banana chunks, along with pomegranate or other juice, to your blender to make a tasty fruit smoothie.

Savoring Sensational Strawberries

Strawberries land on the superfood list because of their terrific nutrition and powerful phytochemicals (plus a low calorie count). They're also a good source of fiber, and strawberries are very sweet, so they don't need extra sugar. These beautiful red berries are the most popular member of the berry family.

Because strawberries are so good for you and fairly inexpensive (compared to other fresh berries), we suggest you enjoy them three or four times a week.

Optimizing health with strawberries

The rich red color in strawberries provides antioxidants, and one cup of strawberry slices gives you more than 100 percent of the vitamin C you need each day for fewer than 50 calories. So strawberries are an excellent food for watching your weight.

Among the health benefits of eating strawberries are the following:

- ✔ **They keep your heart healthy.** Strawberries provide heart-healthy potassium while being low in sodium. Strawberries also contain natural anti-inflammatory agents that may help keep your arteries healthy.

- ✔ **They protect your vision.** Eating three or more servings of fruit every day may help reduce your risk of macular degeneration (the leading cause of blindness in the elderly). The antioxidant lutein may be particularly potent.

- ✔ **They may help prevent cancer and rheumatoid arthritis.** The phenols in strawberries have

powerful anti-cancer properties and may also
prevent rheumatoid arthritis.

✔ **They're natural painkillers.** The phytochemicals
in strawberries are powerful anti-inflammatory
agents that may work to reduce pain similar to
the way ibuprofen and aspirin work — but without the side effects.

✔ **They keep your immune system strong.**
Strawberries contain a lot of vitamin C, which
strengthens your immune system. Vitamin C
also keeps your connective tissue strong for
younger-looking skin.

Selecting, storing, and savoring strawberries

Look for fresh, plump strawberries in the produce
section. Healthy berries should be a rich red in color
and firm to the touch, with no sign of mold or spoil-
age. Strawberries are also available in the frozen
foods section. When you buy frozen strawberries,
read the label to be sure they don't have added sugar.

At home, keep the berries in the refrigerator just as
they are; wait until you're ready to eat them before
you wash them and cut off the stems. Strawberries
are quite perishable, so only buy as many as you
intend to eat over the course of about three days.

When you're ready to use your strawberries, just
rinse them under water and remove the stems.
Strawberries taste delicious whole or sliced and
served in a bowl with a little cream or mixed with
whole-grain cereal. They also work well as an ingredient in fruit smoothies.

Another way to use strawberries is to make a
simple fruit salad by combining strawberry slices,

blueberries, melon chunks, grapes, and pineapple pieces. Strawberries can also be added to a regular garden salad.

Starting the Day with Wholesome Oatmeal

Whole-grain oatmeal has warmed many bellies at breakfast, which may be the most important meal of the day. Whole grains (with the bran and husk intact) are high in fiber, so they're digested more slowly than foods made up of mostly simple carbohydrates (sugars). Whole-grain fiber helps stabilize blood sugar and gives you sustained energy.

Oats have some super benefits to get you ready for the day. They're packed with fiber and other nutrients that are important for your health. We suggest you eat oats at least two times per week.

Exploring the proven benefits of oats

One cup of cooked oats contains 6 grams of protein, 4 grams of fiber, and 166 calories. The type of fiber oatmeal contains seems to be more effective than other types of fiber for lowering cholesterol. Oats also contain polyphenols that fight inflammation and work with vitamin C to keep your blood fats at healthy levels.

Oats also are a good source of minerals like magnesium, manganese, zinc, and selenium. These minerals are important for several chemical reactions that take place in your body, plus selenium is a powerful antioxidant. Oats also contain lutein, a phytochemical related to vitamin A that's important for normal vision.

When you eat oats, you improve your health by

- ✔ Lowering cholesterol
- ✔ Decreasing cardiovascular disease
- ✔ Strengthening your immune system
- ✔ Stabilizing blood sugar

 To make your oatmeal even healthier, add a tablespoon of chia seeds or flax seeds to increase your fiber and add some healthy omega-3 fatty acids. This combination is even more effective in lowering cholesterol and improving heart health than oatmeal alone.

Buying and eating oatmeal

You can find a variety of oats in the cereal section of grocery stores — steel-cut, old-fashioned (rolled), quick-cooking, and instant. Steel-cut oatmeal takes the longest to cook. Old-fashioned oatmeal takes less time because the oats are rolled thin compared to the steel-cut variety. Instant oatmeal has been pre-cooked and is ready almost as soon as you add hot water.

 Read the labels if you buy instant oatmeal. Many brands of instant oatmeal contain excess sugar that you don't need. Look for plain instant oatmeal from reputable brands such as Quaker, and add just a little honey, sweetener, or fresh fruit.

Start your morning with a bowl of hot oatmeal or a whole-grain oat cereal, such as Cheerios. Choose low-fat and low-sugar oatmeal muffins and cookies. Substitute oats for breadcrumbs or part of the wheat flour in some of your recipes.

Chapter 4

Revving Up Your Dishes with Superfoods

In This Chapter

▶ Cooking with olive oil

▶ Incorporating cloves of garlic

▶ Getting nutty with almonds

▶ Cherishing the wonder of chia seeds

*T*rying to incorporate superfoods into your diet may seem overwhelming some days. However, you can sneak superfoods into your favorite standby dishes and hardly notice the difference.

Cook with olive oil instead of butter or vegetable oil, sprinkle almonds or chia seeds onto a salad, or have a piece of garlic bread with dinner or as a snack. You'll be fighting cholesterol, preventing cancer, and watching your weight without a second thought.

This chapter gives you the details on getting superfoods into your diet as unobtrusively as possible.

Pouring It On! Olive Oil

Olive oil is one of the main features of the Mediterranean diet, which appears to be one of the best diets for reducing heart disease risk and living longer.

Olive oil contains *oleic acid* (an omega-9 monounsaturated fat that's good for your health), and virgin and extra virgin olive oils also contain phytochemical antioxidants.

Olives are harvested and taken to mills, where they're cleaned and ground into paste. The oil is separated from the solids and bottled. Oil pressed in this manner is called *virgin* or *extra virgin* olive oil (depending on the oleic acid content). Virgin and extra virgin olive oils are rich in *polyphenols* (natural substances that have health benefits) and have a much better flavor than *refined* olive oil, which has fewer polyphenols than virgin or extra virgin olive oils.

Because olive oil is so good for you and so easy to use, we suggest you consume 2 tablespoons of olive oil every day, preferably in place of saturated animal fats. Don't overdo it, though. Two tablespoons may not seem like much, but oils are high in calories, so a little bit goes a long way.

Reaping the benefits of olive oil

Two tablespoons of olive oil supply 239 calories plus vitamins E and K, monounsaturated fats (which decrease your LDL cholesterol — the bad kind — and raise your HDL cholesterol — the good kind), and polyphenols. These polyphenols, in addition to oleic acid, elevate olive oil from just another healthy food to superfood status.

Olive oil has a positive impact on cholesterol and can help prevent heart disease when you use it to replace unhealthy saturated fats (from such unsuperfoods as fatty red meats and high-fat dairy products, for example).

Adding a little olive oil to your diet imparts several important benefits.

- ✔ **Protecting your heart:** The monounsaturated fats and polyphenols in olive oil help to lower your total cholesterol while raising the good HDL cholesterol. Olive oil also helps to lower blood pressure and keeps your arteries healthy by decreasing inflammation.

- ✔ **Preventing cancer:** Researchers have found that the polyphenols in olive oil may help to reduce the risk of breast cancer by inhibiting the growth of cancer cells and killing H. pylori, bacteria that's been linked to peptic ulcers and stomach cancer.

- ✔ **Longevity:** People who follow a Mediterranean type of diet rich in olive oil, poultry, and vegetables tend to live longer than people who eat more pasta and red meat.

Selecting, storing, and pouring olive oil

Olive oil is available in every market and grocery store. Olive oils vary in price, from refined olive oil, which is the least expensive, to delicately flavored (but not delicately priced) extra virgin olive oils found in exclusive gourmet shops.

Store olive oil in a dark glass bottle or stainless steel container in a cool area, away from any heat sources. You can also store your olive oil in the refrigerator;

however, doing so may alter the flavor of extra virgin olive oil.

You can use olive oil for salad dressings, sauces, and cooking a variety of savory dishes. Here are some ideas:

- ✔ Extra virgin olive oil loses flavor when cooked, so it's better for making dressings or for using on top of cooked foods.

- ✔ Replace butter with olive oil, or blend the two into a spread that has less saturated fat than butter alone.

- ✔ Dip whole-grain bread in olive oil mixed with a little parmesan cheese and red pepper.

- ✔ Dress your salads with extra-virgin olive oil and a bit of balsamic vinegar.

- ✔ Top your cooked vegetables with a drizzle of olive oil and lemon juice.

- ✔ Make pesto using olive oil and serve with pasta.

Livening Up Foods with a Clove of Garlic

Pungent, cream-colored cloves of garlic add more than flavor to your foods; they also bring good health to you and your family.

Garlic has been used as medicine for a very long time to fight infections (not to mention warding off vampires). Today, garlic is used to reduce cholesterol and prevent cancer and as an anti-microbial agent.

Garlic has a distinctive aroma and flavor due to a compound called *allicin,* which is released when the clove is sliced or crushed. Although the heat from cooking reduces some of the active compounds in garlic, cooked garlic still retains most of its health benefits.

We suggest you eat one clove of garlic every day, or take garlic supplements two or three times each week.

Gauging garlic's health benefits

The main active compounds in garlic are allicin and other sulfur-containing compounds.

Garlic also contains some B complex vitamins and selenium, which are important for many chemical reactions in your body. Selenium is a mineral that works like an antioxidant.

Garlic is also very low in calories — one clove has only 4 calories.

You can rely on garlic to assist with the following:

- ✔ Lowering blood pressure
- ✔ Preventing cancer
- ✔ Fighting a variety of fungi, viruses, and bacteria
- ✔ Promoting digestive health

Preparing and using garlic

Fresh garlic is available in the produce section of your grocery store. Garlic is also often available pre-chopped in jars or bottles.

To roast garlic, remove the outermost layer of papery covering and place the bulb in a baking dish. Drizzle some olive oil on top of the bulb, cover the baking dish with aluminum foil, and bake in an oven heated to 375 degrees Fahrenheit for about one hour. Serve the roasted garlic with whole-grain bread.

To prepare garlic for cooking, simply break the cloves you need off the bulb. To make peeling the papery covering off the cloves easier, press down on them with your thumb to crack the "shell" — it's then much easier to peel. Or heat the cloves in your microwave on high for about 10 seconds or so. This loosens the covering. Then chop the peeled cloves with a knife or a garlic press, a device that squeezes the clove through several small holes.

You get the most health benefits from fresh garlic cloves that you chop or crush just before you add them to your recipes. Pre-chopped garlic is not as powerful as fresh garlic; however, it retains much of its health benefit and many people like the convenience. If you choose pre-chopped garlic, buy it in small jars and store the garlic in the refrigerator after it has been opened.

Make garlic bread by first drizzling olive oil on whole-wheat bread, then spreading some roasted garlic on the bread. Top off with a little parmesan cheese, and toast in the oven until golden brown.

Garlic supplements are available at most groceries and health-food stores. Many people prefer taking supplements to avoid the after-effect of "garlic breath." Taking a capsule with an enteric coating diminishes the garlic odor; the coating ensures the garlic is released in the small intestine instead of the stomach.

Adding Almonds to Your Diet

Almonds are crunchy, delicious, and very good for you. They're rich in fiber, monounsaturated fats, and phytochemicals that fight free radicals to keep the cells in your body healthy. You should enjoy almonds whenever you can — just don't think that means you can eat a bunch of Almond Joy candy bars.

Almonds also contain *polyphenols* (phytonutrients that provide health benefits) — especially in the thin brown skin that covers the nut. According to an article published in 2008 in *The Journal of Food Science*, roasting almonds with the skin intact actually concentrates the amount of polyphenols.

We suggest you eat 1 ounce of our superfood nuts every day, such as one serving of almonds (up to 23 nuts).

Filling up on fiber, healthful fats, and antioxidants

Almonds weigh in at 165 calories per ounce. They contain vitamin E and substantial amounts of magnesium, manganese, and copper. Magnesium is involved in many of the biochemical reactions that take place in your body. Manganese is an antioxidant and is necessary for healing wounds and keeping bones strong. Copper is essential for the formation of healthy blood cells.

In addition to all of this, almonds offer the following health benefits:

- ✔ **Lowering cholesterol:** Almonds are rich in *phytosterols* (a plant version of cholesterol that's good for you) that help regulate cholesterol levels in your body. Phytosterols and monounsaturated fats are particularly beneficial when they replace saturated fat, which increases cholesterol.

- ✔ **Preventing anemia:** Almonds supply the mineral copper, which is necessary for normal red blood cell production in your body. Copper and manganese also work as enzymes in some of the chemical reactions in your body that produce energy.

✔ **Easing weight loss:** Although almonds have a lot of calories, substituting monounsaturated fats for saturated fats (found in red meats) may help to increase weight loss, even if you don't cut many calories. Almonds also help keep you full between meals because they're rich in proteins and fiber.

✔ **Protecting your prostate:** A phytosterol found in almonds is effective for decreasing the symptoms of benign prostatic hyperplasia (BPH) in men. BPH is a common condition where the prostate gland enlarges, resulting in difficulty in urination and sexual performance.

✔ **Preventing diabetes:** Almonds slow the rises in blood sugar that occur after eating carbohydrate-rich meals. The polyphenols and vitamin E in almonds also help to protect you from damaging free radicals.

Buying and enjoying almonds

Almonds are easy to find in any grocery store. The best almonds are still in the shells, which protect the delicate fats inside the nuts.

Look for almonds with shells that are unbroken and free of mold.

Use a nutcracker to open almonds. The added effort of cracking the shell makes for automatic portion control because you can't eat them by the handful.

Although fresh almonds are best, they aren't very convenient for cooking. For this purpose, you can find packages of shelled, blanched almonds in the baking section of your grocery store.

You can find roasted almonds in bags or cans in the snack section of the grocery store. Be careful with these almonds, because they're usually roasted in unhealthy oils and contain extra salt and artificial flavorings that may not be good for you.

Store shelled almonds in a covered container in the refrigerator to protect the healthful fats. If you have a large amount (more than you can eat in a week), keep some in the freezer.

You can enjoy a handful of almonds as a protein- and fiber-rich afternoon snack (both protein and fiber will keep you feeling full until dinnertime). Or you can add them to many of your favorite dishes for extra crunch. Almonds have a delicious flavor that works well with savory foods as well as sweet foods.

Here are some delicious ideas for eating almonds:

- ✔ Enjoy almond butter in place of peanut butter on your sandwiches.
- ✔ Eat a handful of almonds with an apple for a superfoods snack.
- ✔ Sprinkle sliced almonds on a salad or on vegetables.
- ✔ Make a yogurt and berry parfait and top it with chopped almonds.
- ✔ Sprinkle slivered almonds over trout.

Discovering Mexico's Chia Seeds

You probably know it best from that fad some years ago called the Chia Pet. Fact is, chia is a superfood.

Chia is a member of the mint family and is native to Mexico, where it has been used for thousands of years in cooking. The ancient Aztecs and Mayans ate chia seeds before entering into battle or making long treks to sustain their energy, give them endurance, and control their appetites when food would be difficult to find.

Chia seeds are very high in omega-3 fatty acids and rich in antioxidants. They are relatively unknown outside of Central America, but they're increasingly gaining recognition as a superfood and, no doubt, demand will grow as the word spreads.

Cashing in on the health benefits of chia

Chia is making a name for itself in nutrition due to its neutral flavor and the fact that it contains large amounts of an omega-3 fatty acid called *alpha-linolenic acid* (ALA). This fatty acid helps your heart and makes it easier to watch your weight.

Chia seeds are rich in calcium, manganese, and fiber, which are important for strong bones and good digestion. Chia contains two antioxidants — *chlorogenic acid* and *caffeic acid* — which are also found in coffee beans.

Chia has a high percentage of protein, and it has all the essential amino acids (the building blocks of protein), so it's a terrific source of protein for vegans.

There are two types of chia: black and white; however, there isn't much difference nutritionally. Both black and white chia seeds offer lots of nutrition. One serving of chia seeds is about 1 ounce and contains 10 grams of fiber and 139 calories.

When you eat chia seeds, you can feel good knowing that you are

✔ **Preventing cardiovascular disease.** Regular chia consumption can lower blood pressure and reduce inflammation. The omega-3 fatty acids are great for lowering cholesterol, which also helps reduce your risk of cardiovascular disease.

✔ **Keeping your gut in check.** The fiber in chia is great for bowel regulation and overall gastrointestinal health. You can also use chia to reduce the pain of heartburn.

✔ **Watching your weight.** Chia helps you feel full longer because it's absorbed and metabolized slowly, which helps regulate *insulin* (a hormone that controls blood sugar), so you won't feel a blood sugar drop that causes hunger.

✔ **Controlling blood sugar.** Because chia is beneficial in regulating insulin, it may aid in treatment of diabetes.

✔ **Getting an energy boost.** Chia seeds can absorb seven to ten times their weight in water, forming a gel that's digested slowly, which helps to keep energy levels high.

Incorporating chia in your diet

Chia seeds are easy to find online, and you may also be able to find them in health food stores.

Store chia seeds at room temperature out of direct sunlight, and they'll keep for up to two years — that's one durable superfood.

You can get your daily dose of chia in several ways. Chia seeds have a neutral flavor, so you can add them to almost any type of food. You can sprinkle chia seeds on cereal or a salad, or stir them into a soup. You can also add them to recipes for bread and muffins.

Alternatively, you can take 1 or 2 tablespoons of chia seeds or chia gel every day as a supplement. Make chia gel by adding 9 ounces of water to 1 ounce of chia seeds, and then mix until a gel forms. Let the gel stand at room temperature for 15 minutes and then store it in the refrigerator. Add the gel to fruit juice or a glass of water, or mix it into your morning bowl of oatmeal. The gel will keep in your refrigerator for up to two weeks.

If you actually *have* a Chia Pet — you know, those clay pots, often in the shape of cartoon characters, that come with a seed-laden paste and sprout a green mini-forest after a couple weeks — don't eat the seeds, even though they're the same. Make sure the chia seeds you buy are packaged as a food product. Chia Pet sprouts aren't approved as a food product by the U.S. Food and Drug Administration (FDA). Get your chia from a local health store.

Chapter 5

Vegging Out in a Good Way

*W*hen you eat a superfoods diet rich in vegetables, you give your body what it needs to stay healthy.

Eating lots of vegetables helps prevent cancer, controls blood pressure, makes weight control much easier, and even keeps your brain healthy. The journal *Neurology* reported in 2006 that diets with lots of vegetables are associated with a slower rate of cognitive decline in the elderly.

You should eat at least four servings of vegetables every day.

Are all vegetables good for your health? Absolutely. Some vegetables, such as potatoes and sweet corn, have gotten a bad reputation with the popularity of low-carbohydrate diets, but they really are healthful vegetables when you prepare them in healthful ways. A baked potato with the skin intact is good for you, for example, but French fries aren't.

Other healthful vegetables include beans, peas, squash, cauliflower, radishes, and greens. These vegetables are all nutrient-dense, which means they have a lot of nutritional value without a lot of calories. So, eating lots of vegetables helps keep you slim.

Although all vegetables are good for you, some are better than others. Some have added benefits from *phytochemicals* (natural compounds found in plants that can improve health and prevent disease) and high concentrations of vitamins, minerals, and fiber. The ones that have these additional benefits are our superfood vegetables.

Superfood vegetables are richly colored with red, orange, and green hues. The pigments in superfood vegetables contain phytochemicals called *flavonoids*, which are powerful antioxidants that fight cell damage in your body.

 Choose vegetables of different colors every day to obtain a variety of phytochemicals that will affect different parts of your body. Dark green and brightly colored vegetables are your best choices to get phytochemicals.

As this chapter explains, superfood vegetables are easy to incorporate into your diet as snacks, side dishes, soups, and salads. Plus they're easy to find in your local grocery stores, many of them store well, and perhaps most important, they taste delicious.

Oh, and be sure to check out Chapters 6 and 7 for some great recipes using superfood veggies.

Dipping into Holy Guacamole: The Avocado

Avocados, like tomatoes, are technically a fruit, but they're usually used in cooking as a vegetable. Avocados have a rough, thick, dark skin that has earned them the nickname "alligator pear." But don't let the tough skin fool you — the flesh inside is smooth, soft, and flavorful due to the avocado's fat content. Avocados are rich in monounsaturated fats that help keep your heart healthy. They're also rich in healthy oils and fiber.

 We suggest that you eat at least one avocado each week.

Making the most of monounsaturated fats

One ounce of avocado (about 2 tablespoons) contains 50 calories and 2 grams of fiber, plus significant amounts of magnesium, potassium, folate, vitamin K, and lutein — quite a lot of nutrition for such a small amount of food.

 Avocados are rich. They have more calories than most vegetables, so be sure to watch your serving sizes. One serving of avocado is only about 2 tablespoons.

Avocados help to keep your heart healthy, reduce the symptoms of an enlarged prostate, and increase your absorption of vitamins A, E, and K. They're good at all of the following:

✔ **Protecting your heart:** Avocados contain *oleic acid,* a heart-healthy monounsaturated fat recommended by the American Heart Association. Oleic acid protects your cardiovascular system by reducing your total cholesterol (elevated levels of cholesterol are linked to an increased risk of heart disease) and increasing your HDL cholesterol (the good kind that helps protect your heart).

Avocados are also a good source of a plant sterol called *beta-sitosterol.* Sterols are found in plant cell membranes and play a role similar to cholesterol in animal cells. Plant sterols lower cholesterol in humans.

The combination of oleic acid, plant sterols, folate, and fiber makes for powerful protection from heart disease.

✔ **Reducing prostate symptoms:** *The British Journal of Urology* reported in 2000 that men who were treated with beta-sitosterol had reduced urinary symptoms due to *benign prostatic hyperplasia,* or enlarged prostates. Follow-up studies found that beta-sitosterol therapy was still effective after 18 months.

✔ **Increasing absorption of fat-soluble vitamins:** Eating fat (the good kind, as in avocados) along with foods containing vitamins A, E, and K helps improve the absorption of those vitamins. Adding a little avocado to a garden salad is a great way to boost vitamin absorption while adding extra nutrition.

Adding avocado to your diet

Fresh avocados are found in the produce section. You can't tell much about an avocado by its tough exterior, but you can tell whether it's ripe by gently squeezing it. A ripe avocado yields just slightly to your touch. It should feel as if it's filled with clay. If it's too soft, you won't be able to slice it, but you can still use it mashed in guacamole or other recipes.

Unripe avocados that are too firm to the touch can be ripened at home. Place them in a brown paper bag and keep them at room temperature for up to five days.

 Your avocados will ripen faster if you place an apple in the bag. Apples give off ethylene gas that speeds ripening fruits and some vegetables.

Avocadoes don't keep very well. Once your avocados are ripe, you can keep them in the refrigerator for only two or three days. So don't buy more avocados than you can use in a couple days.

When you're ready to use an avocado, wash it first to remove any dirt or bacteria. Cut the avocado length-wise around the large seed. Twist the two halves in opposite directions to separate. Slide a spoon under-neath the seed and lift it out. Place the halves cut side down, and peel away the skin. Slice or dice the flesh, and your avocado is ready to go.

You can enjoy avocados on sandwiches, in salads, or as guacamole — a delicious dip made with avocados (see Chapter 6). Add small chunks of avocado to bur-ritos and tacos, too.

Feeling the Beet

Red beets are rich in nutrients and fiber and low in calories, and have a deliciously sweet flavor. Beets also contain antioxidants and other healthy phyto-chemicals. Red beets are often passed over in favor of other, more popular vegetables. That's a real shame,

because they're easy to prepare and extremely good
for you.

We suggest that you eat beets twice each week.

Beating heart disease, birth defects, and metabolic syndrome

The red pigments in beets contain antioxidants called
betalains that may help to reduce risk of heart disease
and other chronic disease.

According to research reported in 2005 in *The Journal
of Agricultural and Food Chemistry,* betalains protect
your body from oxidative stress damage caused by
free radicals. *Free radicals* aren't extremists out on
parole — they're particles that occur as by-products
from normal metabolism and from exposure to
smoke, pollution, or too much sun.

Beets are also rich in a substance called *betaine* that
reduces homocysteine levels (elevated homocysteine
levels correlate with having a higher risk of cardiovascular disease). Betaine may also aid in digestion and
improve your *metabolism,* the rate at which you burn
calories.

Eating two cooked beets gives you 40 calories and
2 grams of fiber, plus magnesium, potassium, and
folate. Beets are also rich in plant sterols. When you
eat beets, you reap the following benefits:

> ✔ **They protect your heart.** The combination of
> folate, fiber, betaine, and sterols helps to pro-
> tect your heart by reducing homocysteine levels
> and keeping cholesterol levels in check. And,
> according to an article published in 2006 in *The
> American Journal of Clinical Nutrition,* betalains
> prevent oxidative damage to blood cholesterol.

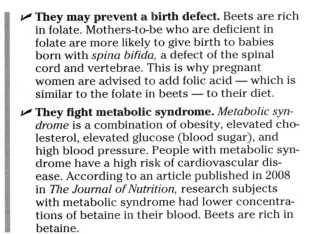

✔ **They may prevent a birth defect.** Beets are rich in folate. Mothers-to-be who are deficient in folate are more likely to give birth to babies born with *spina bifida,* a defect of the spinal cord and vertebrae. This is why pregnant women are advised to add folic acid — which is similar to the folate in beets — to their diet.

✔ **They fight metabolic syndrome.** *Metabolic syndrome* is a combination of obesity, elevated cholesterol, elevated glucose (blood sugar), and high blood pressure. People with metabolic syndrome have a high risk of cardiovascular disease. According to an article published in 2008 in *The Journal of Nutrition,* research subjects with metabolic syndrome had lower concentrations of betaine in their blood. Beets are rich in betaine.

Choosing and enjoying beets

Look for fresh beets in the produce section of your grocery store. They should be a deep red color with smooth skins. Choose small- to medium-sized beets for the best flavor. Avoid beets that have damage to the skin, such as bruising or spots, and pass over those that appear to be dry and shriveled. Store your beets in the refrigerator for up to two weeks.

You can cook red beets and serve them as a side dish, or you can grate raw beets over salads and soups.

To cook beets, first wash the skin gently. Then cut off the greens (which you can use as salad greens), but leave an inch or two of the stem attached to the beets. Don't peel the beets until after they're cooked. Simply boil them until they're tender when you pierce them with a fork.

When you roast vegetables in your oven, add some beets for variety, flavor, and color. You can also purchase heat-and-serve beets in cans or pickled in vinegar.

Eating large quantities of beets may result in pink or reddish-colored urine. Don't be alarmed — this comes from the natural red pigments in beets and is completely harmless.

Betting on Broccoli: A Nutritional Powerhouse

Broccoli is a member of the *cruciferous* family (or mustard family) of vegetables that also includes cauliflower, Brussels sprouts, cabbage, bok choy, and kale (another superfood vegetable — we talk about kale later in this chapter).

Cruciferous vegetables contain several types of natural compounds called *glucosinolates,* which are phytochemicals that have a positive impact on your health by reducing your risk of cancer. Broccoli is a superfood vegetable because it contains both glucosinolates and large amounts of other nutrients that are crucial for good health.

The dark green pigment of broccoli contains antioxidant phytochemicals along with several vitamins, such as vitamins A, K, and C.

Broccoli is such a nutritional powerhouse that we suggest you eat broccoli (either raw or cooked) four times each week.

Providing a wealth of health benefits

One cup of chopped broccoli gives you a full day's supply of vitamin C, a water-soluble vitamin that your body can't store and therefore needs to replace frequently. Vitamin C keeps your immune system strong so you can fight colds, flu, and infections. Vitamin C also protects your skin by keeping the underlying connective tissue strong.

Broccoli contains lots of vitamins A and K — two fat-soluble vitamins that are important for normal vision, healthy cell growth, and normal blood clotting.

Eating broccoli also provides you with calcium, potassium, and magnesium. These minerals keep your bones strong and are necessary for your muscles and nerves to work normally.

Finally, broccoli is a great source of fiber (1 cup contains 3 grams), which is good for your digestive system and cholesterol levels. And because 1 cup of broccoli contains a mere 30 calories, you can eat large portions of broccoli with no negative impact on your weight.

And as if all these benefits weren't enough, broccoli enhances your health in the following ways, too:

> ✔ **Preventing cancer:** Broccoli has been found to be effective in preventing several types of cancer, including prostate, bladder, colon, breast, and ovarian cancers. In fact, in 1994 *The American Journal of Clinical Nutrition* reported findings that broccoli was the best vegetable for preventing colon cancer.
>
> According to the American Cancer Society, this anti-cancer action may be attributable to the fact that the phytochemicals in broccoli boost detoxifying enzymes.

Researchers also believe that two important glucosinolates found in broccoli — *sulphorophane* and *indole-3-carbonyl* — play a starring role. In particular, indole-3 carbonyl has been shown to prevent breast and ovarian cancers.

✔ **Promoting clear vision as you age:** Your eyes contain substantial amounts of lutein and zeaxanthin, two phytochemicals related to vitamin A that are also found in the dark green pigments of broccoli. The journal *Archives of Ophthalmology* reported in 2007 that people who consume diets that were rich in lutein and zeaxanthin were less likely to suffer from macular degeneration, a deterioration of eyesight associated with aging.

✔ **Maintaining cardiovascular health:** The effect of lutein on the heart is similar to that of aspirin — without the side effects. The lutein in broccoli acts as an anti-inflammatory agent that reduces plaque in your blood vessels, most importantly the arteries that feed your heart. Plaque build-up leads to *atherosclerosis* (a narrowing of the arteries), reduces blood flow to vital organs, and increases your risk for heart attacks and strokes. Broccoli fights that.

The folate found in broccoli helps to keep homocysteine levels low (high levels are associated with heart disease), and its potassium helps to keep blood pressure normal. As an added benefit, broccoli is low in sodium, an important consideration if you're watching your blood pressure.

✔ **Preventing a birth defect:** The risk for spina bifida is higher when mothers-to-be don't get enough folate in their diets, especially during the initial stages of pregnancy. Broccoli, along with other dark green vegetables, is a good source of folate.

Buying, storing, and preparing broccoli

Fresh broccoli is available in the produce department of every grocery store.

Look for dark green, tightly packed florets (the darker the green tint, the more phytonutrients it contains). The stem should not be woody, and the leaves should not be wilted. You can also buy frozen broccoli, either alone or combined with other vegetables. You can even find broccoli sprouts in some stores.

 Some frozen broccoli products include seasonings or sauces. Some sauces are light and healthy, but others are high in calories and sodium, so be sure to read Nutrition Facts labels before you buy frozen broccoli (or any frozen vegetables for that matter).

Broccoli keeps well in the refrigerator. Store broccoli in the vegetable drawer and use it within a few days. Wash the broccoli just before you prepare it, not before you put it in the fridge. Cut the florets off the stem and break into bite-sized pieces. Slice the stem into similar-sized chunks.

 You can eat both the florets and the stem; however, broccoli stems take longer to cook.

Broccoli can be steamed or boiled, but don't overcook it: Florets only need about five minutes. The stems need another minute or two.

Broccoli also works well in stir-fry dishes. Add stem pieces to hot oil and stir for one minute before adding the florets, and cook everything for another minute or so. Broccoli is done when it is crisp-tender and very bright green. It also produces an intense, good smell when it's done.

Serve crunchy raw broccoli pieces with veggie dip or salad dressing, or add them to garden salads and side dishes. See Chapter 7 for delicious and healthy broccoli recipes.

 Use broccoli sprouts in salads or on sandwiches, just as you would use alfalfa sprouts.

Cutting Heart Disease with Carrots

Carrots are delicious any time of year. Bright orange carrots contain lots of vitamin A, which helps keep your vision healthy, and antioxidants plus phytonutrients that may help to prevent cancer.

Carrots are high in fiber and low in calories, so they're good for weight-loss diets. Bugs Bunny had the right idea, but you definitely don't need to be a rabbit to enjoy nibbling on fresh carrots.

Carrots are versatile and very nutritious whether you enjoy them as a raw crunchy snack or cooked as a side dish.

 We suggest you eat carrots two to three times each week.

Exploiting carotenes and phytochemicals

Carrots have lots of vitamin A, a substantial amount of vitamin C (about 10 percent of what you need for one day), and a lot of beta carotene.

One cup of carrots contains 20,381 International Units of vitamin A, which is six times the amount you need for the day!

Vitamin A has many health benefits:

- ✔ It sharpens your eyesight because a form of vitamin A called *retinal* is important in the retinas of your eyes.
- ✔ It triggers production of white blood cells that fight infection.
- ✔ It promotes normal cell growth and reproduction.

Vitamin C is important for strong immune system function and in forming strong connective tissue under your skin, which helps, believe it or not, to prevent wrinkles.

Beta carotene is a powerful antioxidant that protects your cells and keeps you young. Carrots are also a good source of niacin (a B vitamin), potassium, and calcium.

Other benefits you can take advantage of by eating carrots include the following:

- ✔ **Preventing certain cancers:** A 2008 article in *Nutrition and Cancer* stated that diets rich in carotenoids (beta carotene, lutein, and zeaxanthin — all related to vitamin A) are associated with a lower risk of cervical cancer in women.

  Research published in 2005 in *The Journal of Agricultural and Food Chemistry* found that a phytochemical found in carrots called falcarinol prevented cancer in lab rats.

- ✔ **Preventing diabetes:** Research published in 2008 in the journal *Diabetes Care* confirms that high levels of carotenoids in the blood are associated with a lower risk of diabetes. Eating a healthy diet, watching your weight, and getting the carotenoids found in carrots can help prevent the onset of type II diabetes (which most often occurs in adults).

✔ **Helping you lose weight:** One cup of sliced carrots contains only 50 calories, plus lots of fiber, so eating carrots is a great way to feed your craving for crunchy foods while you're watching your weight.

Finding and preparing carrots

You can find carrots in the fresh produce section, the canned foods section, and the freezer section of the grocery store. You can also use carrots as ingredients in soups, salads, and slaws.

Canned carrots often lack the flavor of fresh or frozen carrots, but they're convenient. Be sure to read the label to avoid excess sodium.

As for fresh carrots, choose ones that are bright orange and firm. Avoid fresh carrots that are soft or appear to be shriveled.

Store carrots in the vegetable crisper in your refrigerator. Carrots keep well for about two weeks as long as they're not cut. After they're peeled and cut, they should be eaten within three or four days.

Add extra chunks of carrots to soups and stews, or grate a carrot on top of a salad. Serve our ginger-glazed carrots (see Chapter 7) as a sweet side dish that even picky eaters will enjoy.

Chapter 6

Superfood Breakfasts, Snacks, Appetizers, and Desserts

In This Chapter

▶ Understanding why you need to eat breakfast

▶ Making breakfast quick and easy

▶ Indulging on weekends

▶ Snacking on sensational superfoods

▶ Serving superfoods starters

▶ Dressing up your desserts

*1*s eating breakfast all that important? Yes, absolutely. Kids who've eaten breakfast have an easier time learning in school, and people who eat breakfast every day have an easier time watching their weight. This doesn't mean that just any food will do. A couple of glazed donuts with a can of high-caffeine soda isn't a good breakfast. Cold cereal from a box is better, but still may have too much sugar. There are much healthier alternatives, and breakfast time is a great time to start with some superfoods.

You may think it isn't possible to eat snacks, appetizers, and desserts that are both delicious and healthy for you. Actually, these items also offer a great way to incorporate superfoods into your day.

In this chapter, we give you some delicious and easy breakfast ideas, tips, and recipes so you can start every day with a super breakfast. We also provide some tips on choosing and preparing easy snacks, appetizers, and desserts, as well as the best ways to get the most superfoods in each portion. And of course we offer a some healthy *and* yummy recipes to try out.

Understanding the Most Important Meal of the Day

When you eat breakfast, you *break* the *fast* your body went through during the night. You need breakfast to refuel your body and your brain. A study reported in the journal *Pediatrics* found that high school students who eat breakfast are more alert and have better cognitive function. The same goes for adults, too. When you eat breakfast, you replenish the glucose (a type of sugar) that your brain needs to function, so you feel better and think better.

Unfortunately, many people mistakenly believe that skipping breakfast will help them lose weight, but it doesn't work. According to the Mayo Clinic, eating breakfast is actually good for weight loss. People who eat breakfast every day are much *more* likely to be at a healthy weight. When you skip breakfast, you end up eating too much when you do finally eat.

That doesn't mean you have to eat the instant you get out of bed. You can wait to eat until you feel hungry. Just remember to eat something nutritious.

Not any old breakfast will do. You need to eat a healthful, balanced breakfast to start your day. Choose a variety of foods that will give you plenty of nutrients and fiber, such as whole grains, low-fat dairy products, protein sources, and fruits and vegetables. Here are some examples of simple but healthful breakfasts:

- ✔ A slice of whole-grain toast with almond butter, a fresh piece of fruit, and a glass of nonfat milk

- ✔ A small bowl of whole-grain, high-fiber cold cereal with blueberries and nonfat milk, and calcium-fortified orange juice

- ✔ One hard-boiled egg, a small whole-grain bagel, and low-fat cream cheese with a cup of green tea

- ✔ Hot oatmeal topped with strawberries and walnuts

Making Super Breakfast Recipes

When you add superfoods to your breakfast lineup, you take breakfast to a higher level. Breakfast is a super time to get these superfoods into your day:

- ✔ **Oats:** Enjoy oatmeal, whole-grain bread, muffins, or cereal, or add oats to pancake and waffle recipes.

- ✔ **Fruits and berries:** A piece of fresh fruit, such as an apple, banana, or orange, can be added to any breakfast. Sliced fruits and berries can be added to cereal or to crepes, pancakes, or waffles.

- ✔ **Nuts and seeds:** Top oatmeal with walnuts, pecans, or almonds, or sprinkle flax or chia seeds on your cereal.

> ✔ **Green tea:** Replace one cup of coffee with hot green tea.
>
> ✔ **Vegetables:** Include spinach, broccoli, or tomatoes in egg dishes.

The following recipes can help you get some of these superfoods in your breakfast. We have "breakfast-on-the-go" recipes for foods that you can grab just before you head out the door. We also have some easy recipes that take a little more time, but not much effort. They'll be ready about the same time your coffee's done. There are also delicious recipes that are perfect for weekends or whenever you have a little extra time.

Eating on the go

These recipes are perfect for anyone who has a habit of skipping breakfast because "there just isn't enough time." Breakfast doesn't need to be a full-sized, sit-down meal, with lots of dirty pots, pans, and dishes to wash.

The secret is to have your breakfast foods ready to go so they don't need much preparation. Make our muffins or granola on the weekends and use them for breakfast during the week. Your breakfast-on-the-go items may also include hard-boiled eggs, whole-wheat toast with nut butter, and single-serving cups of yogurt (but avoid extra sugar).

Some of our superfood breakfast recipes may not be as sweet as the cereal and pastry items you may be used to eating. But cutting back on sugar allows you to taste the flavors of the fruits, nuts, and grains. If you're used to a sugary breakfast, you can add a little sugar, honey, 100 percent fruit spread or artificial sweetener — just not too much.

Oatmeal Blueberry Muffins

Make these muffins the night before, so they're ready to go in the morning. These muffins aren't as sweet as the muffins you find in bakeries and coffee shops, but they're delicious plain. You can also spread a little 100 percent fruit spread or honey on them for extra flavor and sweetness. These muffins are healthy because they incorporate two superfoods — blueberries and oatmeal — and because they're 100 percent whole-grain.

Prep time: *About 10 minutes*

Cooking time: *25 minutes*

Yield: *8 servings*

¾ cup whole-wheat flour

¾ cup old-fashioned rolled oats

¼ cup firmly packed dark brown sugar

1½ teaspoons baking powder

½ teaspoon salt

½ cup plain nonfat yogurt

¼ cup low-fat or nonfat milk

2 tablespoons canola oil

1 large egg, beaten lightly

¾ cup fresh or frozen blueberries

1 Preheat oven to 400 degrees Fahrenheit.

2 In a bowl, stir together the flour, oats, brown sugar, baking powder, and salt.

3 In second bowl, combine the yogurt, milk, oil, and egg. Stir the yogurt mixture into the flour mixture until just combined. Fold in blueberries.

4 Divide the batter among 8 paper-lined cupcake tins and bake on the middle rack of oven for 25 minutes.

Per serving: *Calories 152 (From Fat 45); Fat 5g (Saturated 1g); Cholesterol 27mg; Sodium 245mg; Carbohydrate 23g (Dietary Fiber 3g); Protein 5g.*

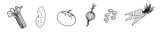

⬭ *Make-Your-Own Granola*

Make this granola to keep handy as a quick snack, or eat it as a cold cereal with milk. This granola has a toasty, nutty flavor and is a delicious way to enjoy almonds, oats, and cranberries.

Prep time: About 10 minutes

Cooking time: 20 to 30 minutes

Yield: 6 servings

2 cups rolled oats	¼ cup raw unsalted pumpkin seeds
½ cup raw unsalted slivered almonds	¼ cup honey
¼ cup raw unsalted sunflower seeds	½ cup canola oil
	½ cup dried cranberries

1 Preheat oven to 300 degrees Fahrenheit.

2 Mix together oats, almonds, and sunflower and pumpkin seeds in a bowl.

3 Mix the honey and oil together in a separate bowl, then pour onto dry mixture. Stir well.

4 Spread onto a greased baking pan and bake for 20 to 30 minutes, or until golden in color, stirring occasionally.

5 Pour into bowl and add cranberries. Let the granola cool, then store in a covered container.

6 At breakfast time, pour ¾ cup cereal into bowl and add milk, or pack in individual snack bags.

Per serving: Calories 458 (From Fat 275); Fat 31g (Saturated 3g); Cholesterol 0mg; Sodium 3mg; Carbohydrate 42g (Dietary Fiber 5g); Protein 9g.

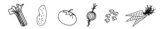

🍂 Simple Peanut Butter and Banana Smoothie

Smoothies are delicious and very good for you when you use healthful ingredients. This breakfast smoothie is a good source of protein and is super with the addition of the banana. You could make it even more super by using plain soy beverage instead of milk.

Prep time: *About 5 minutes*

Yield: *1 serving*

1 banana (for best texture, peel, break into chunks, and freeze ahead of time)

⅔ cup low-fat or nonfat milk

2 tablespoons peanut butter

1 tablespoon honey

3 to 4 ice cubes

1 Combine banana, milk, peanut butter, and honey in blender. Blend at high speed until smooth and creamy.

2 Add ice and blend until smooth. Pour in a tall glass to serve.

Per serving: *Calories 431 (From Fat 168); Fat 19g (Saturated 5g); Cholesterol 7mg; Sodium 235mg; Carbohydrate 59g (Dietary Fiber 5g); Protein 15g.*

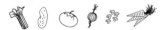

Ready-to-eat cereals

Grocery stores devote entire aisles to ready-to-eat cereals that are convenient and tasty, and some are quite healthful. Just about all cereals are fortified with extra vitamins and minerals. The problem is that some are overloaded with sugar, especially kids' cereals. Too much sugar means too many calories. Read the labels. Choose cereals that are low in sugar (even the non-frosted cereals can be sugary) and high in fiber. Look for the words "100 percent whole wheat" or "100 percent whole grain" on the label. Shredded wheat, toasted oat rings, and puffed wheat bran flakes are all excellent choices. Dress them up with berries, sliced bananas, raisins, or peaches. Need a little more sweetness? Add one teaspoon of sugar or honey, or a little sucralose (Splenda).

Easy breakfast recipes

Maybe you aren't in a big rush in the morning, but you still don't want to spend time cooking extravagant breakfast foods. Not to worry. These recipes are easy to make and taste great.

These recipes feature fresh fruits that are rich in nutrients and fiber, plus whole grains whenever possible. Oats are our favorite whole grain, and we also include a recipe for hot quinoa, which is perfect to warm up with on a cold morning.

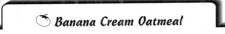

🍠 *Banana Cream Oatmeal*

A bowl of hot oatmeal is so good on a cool morning. Oatmeal is already a superfood, but we add a banana to make it even more super. This is a little sweeter than our other breakfast recipes, so it's a great choice for kids (or grown-ups) who have grown accustomed to sugary breakfast cereals.

Prep time: *About 2 minutes*

Cooking time: *4 minutes*

Yield: *2 servings*

1 cup rolled oats	*½ cup banana slices*
1¾ cups water	*2 tablespoons half-and-half (or substitute nonfat milk, soy beverage, or rice milk)*
1 tablespoon brown sugar (or substitute artificial sweetener)	
	¼ cup walnuts (optional)
⅛ teaspoon salt	

1 Stir the oats, water, brown sugar, and salt together in a microwave-safe bowl.

2 Microwave on high for 2 minutes. Remove from microwave, add bananas and stir. Return to microwave and cook for additional 2 minutes.

3 Divide oatmeal into two serving bowls. Drizzle with half-and-half and top with walnuts if desired.

Per serving: *Calories 234 (From Fat 40); Fat 4g (Saturated 2g); Cholesterol 6mg; Sodium 156mg; Carbohydrate 43g (Dietary Fiber 5g); Protein 7g.*

☕ Fruit and Yogurt Parfait

This beautiful breakfast packs a nutritional punch with fresh fruit, yogurt, and granola. The recipe is versatile, too. You can choose one type of fruit or use a mixture of different fruits and berries. Use our Make-Your-Own Granola (see the preceding section) or any whole-grain cereal.

Prep time: *About 5 to 10 minutes*

Yield: *2 servings*

1 cup plain nonfat yogurt

¼ cup honey (optional)

1 cup fresh cherries, strawberries, blueberries (or these fruits can be frozen,

thawed, and drained) and/or banana slices

½ cup granola or whole-grain cereal

1 Mix yogurt and honey in a small mixing bowl.

2 Spoon half of the fruit or berries into the bottom of each parfait glass.

3 Add half of the yogurt to each glass.

4 Top with half of the granola or cereal.

Per serving: *Calories 233 (From Fat 47); Fat 5g (Saturated 2g); Cholesterol 3mg; Sodium 104mg; Carbohydrate 39g (Dietary Fiber 3g); Protein 10g.*

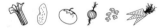

Strawberry Breakfast Pizzas

Fresh strawberries are rich in vitamin C and phyto-chemicals that help to keep you healthy, and they're the featured ingredient in this breakfast pizza recipe. This is very easy to make and fun for kids to assemble with a little help.

Prep time: *About 10 minutes*

Yield: *4 servings*

2 whole-wheat English muffins

⅓ cup plain nonfat yogurt

1 tablespoon honey

¾ cup fresh strawberries, sliced (frozen strawberries may be too soft and mushy)

2 tablespoons strawberry all-fruit spread

1 Split and toast English muffins.

2 In a small bowl, mix together the yogurt and honey.

3 Spoon ¼ of the yogurt and honey mixture onto each English muffin half. Place a layer of strawberry slices on each half.

4 Warm the fruit spread in the microwave oven in 5-second bursts (up to 15 seconds), until it's similar in consistency to syrup.

5 Drizzle the warm fruit spread over the muffins and serve.

Per serving: *Calories 125 (From Fat 8); Fat 1g (Saturated 0g); Cholesterol 0mg; Sodium 228mg; Carbohydrate 27g (Dietary Fiber 3g); Protein 4g.*

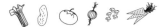

☙ Hot Quinoa with Cinnamon and Fruit

Quinoa is actually a seed, but we use it like a grain in cooking. It has a light fluffy texture and a slightly nutty flavor. In this recipe, we combine quinoa with berries and bananas for a hot breakfast dish that's high in fiber and nutrients.

Prep time: *About 10 minutes*

Cooking time: *About 15 minutes*

Yield: *4 servings*

1 cup nonfat milk	*½ cup bananas*
1 cup water	*½ teaspoon ground cinnamon*
1 cup quinoa, rinsed	
1½ cups fresh blueberries and/or strawberries	*2 tablespoons honey*
	Pinch of salt

1 Combine milk, water, and quinoa in saucepan. Bring to a boil over high heat.

2 Reduce heat to low, cover, and simmer for about 15 minutes, or until most of the liquid is absorbed.

3 Remove from heat and let stand for 5 minutes. Stir in berries, bananas, and cinnamon.

4 Serve immediately in four bowls. Add a drizzle of honey and pinch of salt to each bowl.

Tip: Instead of fresh berries, you can use frozen blue-berries, thawed and drained, but frozen strawberries may be too mushy and should be avoided.

Per serving: *Calories 229 (From Fat 26); Fat 3g (Saturated 0g); Cholesterol 1mg; Sodium 44mg; Carbohydrate 45g (Dietary Fiber 5g); Protein 8g.*

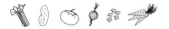

Living lavishly on the weekends

Start your weekend mornings with these healthful and delicious breakfast recipes that are worth the little extra time they take to prepare. These are recipes that will satisfy your sweet tooth (with less sugar) plus two savory egg dishes. We've cut back the sugar and brought out the flavor of the fruits. Our egg dishes contain superfood vegetables and nuts. Don't want to eat eggs? Our egg dishes will work with substitutes such as Egg Beaters.

The lowdown on natural sweeteners

What is the nutritional difference between regular sugar and high-fructose corn syrup? *Almost nothing.* What about between regular sugar and turbinado (raw sugar)? *Just the color.* What about honey — is that better? *Maybe a little, but very little.* Nutritionally, honey and sugar are the same. Some experts claim some honey has some health benefits, but research to support those claims isn't clear. What is clear, though, is the delicious flavor of honey. But don't give honey to children under 1 year of age, as it can cause botulism in babies.

Americans really like sweet stuff. Sodas, candies, and pastries are obviously high in sugar, but sugar is creeping into lots of processed foods. According to the U.S. Department of Agriculture, consumption of sweeteners in processed foods has gone up 23 percent since the 1980s, resulting in increased calorie intakes. Combine that with less physical activity, and the result is unwanted weight gain that leads to chronic diseases such as heart disease, diabetes, and some cancers.

Does this mean you should eliminate all sweeteners from your diet? No. A small amount of sugar or honey or even high-fructose corn syrup every day is okay. Just be aware of what you eat. Read labels, opt for whole foods, and choose recipes wisely.

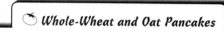

Whole-Wheat and Oat Pancakes

Homemade pancakes are a favorite breakfast food, but typical pancakes are low in fiber and high in sugar. These pancakes are better for you because they're made with whole grains and nonfat milk and have the additional goodness of applesauce.

Prep time: *About 10 minutes*

Cooking time: *About 4 minutes for each pancake*

Yield: *4 servings*

1 egg	½ cup unsweetened applesauce
½ cup oat flour	
½ cup whole-wheat flour	2 tablespoons canola oil
½ cup nonfat milk	2 teaspoons baking powder
	Canola oil or nonstick cooking spray

1 Whisk the egg in mixing bowl until beaten.

2 Add flours, milk, applesauce, oil, and baking powder; mix well.

3 Heat skillet over medium heat and coat with oil or nonstick cooking spray.

4 Pour ¼ cup of batter into skillet, cook until batter bubbles, about two minutes, turn and cook for two more minutes.

5 Repeat for the rest of the batter.

6 Serve with light syrup or fruit spread.

Per serving: *Calories 201 (From Fat 84); Fat 9g (Saturated 1g); Cholesterol 54mg; Sodium 223mg; Carbohydrate 24g (Dietary Fiber 4g); Protein 7g.*

❦ *Cinnamon Blueberry Whole-Grain Waffles*

These waffles include oats and blueberries to make them into superfood waffles. We also use whole-wheat flour for a hearty flavor and more fiber.

Prep time: *About 15 minutes*

Cooking time: *About 5 minutes for each waffle*

Yield: *8 servings*

1¼ cup whole-wheat flour	*1½ cups reduced-fat milk*
½ cup quick-cooking oats	*2 tablespoons canola oil*
3 teaspoons baking powder	*1 large egg, lightly beaten*
¼ teaspoon salt	*1 cup fresh blueberries, or frozen blueberries, thawed and drained*
½ teaspoon cinnamon	

1 Heat waffle iron following manufacturer's instructions.

2 In a large bowl, combine flour, oats, baking powder, salt, and cinnamon.

3 In a separate bowl, stir together milk, canola oil, and egg.

4 Combine wet and dry ingredients and stir until large lumps disappear (don't over-mix).

5 Fold in blueberries.

6 Make waffles according to your waffle iron's instructions. Serve with light syrup or nonfat whipped topping and more blueberries.

Per serving: *Calories 153 (From Fat 48); Fat 5g (Saturated 1g); Cholesterol 28mg; Sodium 249mg; Carbohydrate 22g (Dietary Fiber 3g); Protein 6g.*

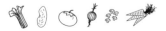

⌣ *Blueberry Yogurt Crepes*

These crepes are made with whole-wheat flour, yet they're still nice and light. The filling is made with yogurt and honey for a sweet and tangy flavor that goes nicely with blueberries. Don't have any blueberries? Try strawberries instead.

Prep time: *About 15 minutes*

Cooking time: *About 2 minutes for each crepe*

Yield: *4 servings (2 crepes each)*

1 cup low-fat milk	1 cup plain nonfat yogurt
¾ cup whole-wheat flour	2 tablespoons honey
2 eggs	¼ teaspoon vanilla
¼ teaspoon salt	1½ to 2 cups fresh blueberries or frozen blueberries, thawed and drained
Canola oil or nonstick cooking spray	

1 Combine milk, flour, eggs, and salt. Whisk until smooth.

2 Heat a nonstick 11-inch skillet over medium heat, and then spray it with nonstick spray or swipe with an oiled paper towel.

3 Pour ¼ cup crepe batter into the skillet. Pick up the skillet and swirl it around gently to spread the batter. Cook for 40 seconds.

4 Carefully turn crepe over and cook for another 40 seconds. Repeat for each crepe, remembering to spray or oil the skillet again.

5 Combine yogurt, honey, and vanilla in mixing bowl and blend thoroughly.

6 Spoon about 1 tablespoon of yogurt mixture and ¼ cup blueberries onto each crepe. Roll and serve.

Per serving: *Calories 237 (From Fat 35); Fat 4g (Saturated 1g); Cholesterol 110mg; Sodium 260mg; Carbohydrate 41g (Dietary Fiber 4g); Protein 12g.*

⟡ Spinach Quiche with Pecans

Quiche is a Sunday brunch staple, although many think it's high in fat and calories. Our version has less cheese, no high-fat crust, and no greasy bacon, and includes the superfoods spinach and pecans.

Prep time: *About 20 minutes*

Cooking time: *About 40 to 45 minutes*

Yield: *4 servings*

Nonstick cooking spray

4 eggs

1 onion, chopped

10-ounce package frozen chopped spinach, thawed and drained

½ cup grated Monterey Jack cheese

½ cup grated Parmesan cheese

½ cup low-fat cottage cheese

⅓ cup chopped pecans

½ teaspoon salt

¼ teaspoon ground black pepper

⅛ teaspoon ground nutmeg

1 Preheat oven to 325 degrees Fahrenheit.

2 Spray a 9-inch glass pie pan with nonstick cooking spray.

3 Add eggs to mixing bowl; whisk until beaten. Mix in the rest of the ingredients, and pour into pie pan.

4 Bake for 35 to 40 minutes, or until a knife inserted into center of the quiche comes out clean.

Per serving: *Calories 293 (From Fat 180); Fat 20g (Saturated 7g); Cholesterol 234mg; Sodium 798mg; Carbohydrate 9g (Dietary Fiber 3g); Protein 21g.*

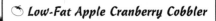

Low-Fat Apple Cranberry Cobbler

Apples and cranberries are two of our superfood fruits, and this apple cranberry cobbler can be breakfast or a delicious dessert. Leave the peelings on your apples for extra nutrition and fiber.

Prep time: *About 20 minutes*

Cooking time: *About 25 to 30 minutes*

Yield: *8 servings*

3 apples, cored and cut into bite-sized chunks	*¾ cup whole-wheat flour*
	½ cup rolled oats
½ cup fresh cranberries or frozen cranberries, thawed and drained	*1½ teaspoon baking powder*
	1 teaspoon sugar
½ cup honey	*¼ teaspoon salt*
¼ cup water or apple juice	*⅔ cup skim milk*
½ teaspoon cinnamon	*2 tablespoons canola oil*
¼ teaspoon nutmeg	*Nonstick cooking spray*

1 Preheat oven to 325 degrees Fahrenheit.

2 Place apples, cranberries, honey, water or apple juice, cinnamon, and nutmeg in a saucepan and cook over medium heat until apples are tender and cranberries pop and open, about 20 minutes.

3 In a mixing bowl, blend flour, oats, baking powder, sugar, and salt.

4 Add milk and canola oil to the dry mixture; stir just until dry ingredients are moistened.

5 Spray a 9-inch pie plate with nonstick spray and fill it with warm apple mixture.

6 Drop dough by spoonfuls onto top of apple mixture, covering evenly.

7 Bake in oven for 25 to 30 minutes, until topping is golden brown.

Per serving: Calories 143 (From Fat 17); Fat 2g (Saturated 0g); Cholesterol 0mg; Sodium 156mg; Carbohydrate 31g (Dietary Fiber 4g); Protein 3g.

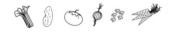

🍅 Vegetable Omelet

Enjoy this omelet for breakfast served with whole-grain toast and a glass of orange juice. It contains garlic and tomatoes as superfoods, and other healthful vegetables.

Prep time: *About 15 minutes*

Cooking time: *About 7 to 8 minutes*

Yield: *4 servings*

3 eggs (or equivalent egg substitute, such as Egg Beaters)

¼ cup nonfat milk

Canola oil or nonstick cooking spray

3 green onions, chopped

1 clove garlic, chopped

¼ cup mushrooms

¼ cup chopped red or green pepper

¼ chopped tomato without seeds

¼ cup grated cheddar cheese

Salt and black pepper to taste

1 Whisk eggs and milk in mixing bowl.

2 Spray nonstick skillet with nonstick cooking spray, or coat lightly with canola oil. Heat over medium heat.

3 Add onions, garlic, mushrooms, peppers, and tomatoes to the skillet and cook until onions are translucent, stirring continuously.

4 Transfer vegetables to a bowl. Wipe the skillet and re-apply nonstick spray or oil.

5 Add eggs to the skillet. As the eggs cook, loosen the edges and let the raw egg slide underneath. Cook for about 1 minute.

6 When eggs appear nearly cooked, add onions, garlic, mushrooms, peppers, tomatoes, cheese, salt, and black pepper to half of the omelet.

7 Fold the other side of the omelet over the filling. Turn off heat and cover. Serve after the cheese is melted, about one minute.

Per serving: Calories 98 (From Fat 48); Fat 5g (Saturated 2g); Cholesterol 163mg; Sodium 290mg; Carbohydrate 5g (Dietary Fiber 1g); Protein 8g.

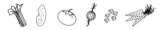

Satisfying Snacking with Superfoods

Many people who want to lose weight believe that snacking is their biggest problem. They think that snacking automatically means eating too much. The truth is that snacking can be good for you. Eating snacks throughout the day can help regulate your body's insulin response and control cravings.

It's not snacking that causes you to gain weight; it's the foods that you choose to snack on. Snacking can actually be a great way to watch your weight when you choose the right foods.

Many superfoods make the simplest, healthiest snacks in their natural, whole state. What could be easier than grabbing an apple from your fruit bowl, munching on a handful of mixed nuts, or dipping broccoli pieces into your favorite veggie dip?

 When you combine two or more superfoods, you can use their different flavors and textures to satisfy cravings without ruining your healthy superfoods diet. The following are a few delicious examples:

✔ **Apples and almond butter:** Slice up a sweet-tangy apple, like a Gala, and serve with a little almond butter. The apple gives you crunchy and sweet, while the almond butter gives you savory, smooth, and just a little salt. Of course, if you don't have almond butter, you can use peanut butter and still get good nutrition.

✔ **Mixed berries with whipped topping and nuts:** Another great combination is a mix of fresh blueberries, strawberries, and raspberries with a dollop of low-calorie whipped topping and a sprinkling of walnuts or pecans. This is just as delicious as a fattening ice cream sundae and so much better for you.

✔ **Veggies and dip:** Raw vegetables can not only tame your craving for savory foods, but because superfood vegetables are loaded with fiber, they also keep you feeling full. Dip some carrot slices into your favorite salad dressing. Or, instead of regular chip dip, dip some baked chips into tomato salsa or guacamole.

Super Snack, Appetizer, and Dessert Recipes

Superfoods make great snacks just as they are, but we know there are times when you want something more. Maybe you need a great appetizer to take to a party, or maybe you just want something new to snack on. In that case, you've come to the right place. Here are some recipes for delicious snacks, appetizers, and desserts that feature superfoods, so you can serve healthy snacks to your family and make delicious desserts that won't bust your diet.

Snacking on superfoods

Snacks are great for tiding you over until your next meal. Here are some recipes that are easy to make when you need a little something to eat and it's not quite lunch or dinnertime.

○ Strawberry Mocha Smoothie

Fruit smoothies have become wildly popular, but many of the ones you buy at coffee shops are made from mixes and don't even contain any real fruit. Make this deliciously healthy berry mocha smoothie at home.

Prep time: *About 10 minutes*

Yield: *2 servings*

½ cup cold coffee (brewed strong)

¼ cup milk

3 tablespoons unsweetened cocoa powder (not Dutch processed)

¼ teaspoon cinnamon

2 teaspoons sugar or sucralose

1 banana, frozen and cut into 1-inch pieces

4 large strawberries

½ cup ice cubes

1 Pour coffee and milk into electric blender. Add cocoa powder, cinnamon, and sucralose. Blend on high speed for 10 seconds.

2 Add the banana, strawberries, and ice cubes and blend on high speed until smooth.

Per serving: Calories 181 (From Fat 29); Fat 3g (Saturated 2g); Cholesterol 4mg; Sodium 20mg; Carbohydrate 42g (Dietary Fiber 7g); Protein 5g.

🍅 Chia Fruit Smoothie

This chia smoothie makes a great snack. The chia seed can absorb ten times its weight, so it has a strong filling effect and a sustained release of energy. Of the plant-based superfoods, chia also has one of the highest concentrations of omega-3 and omega-6 fatty acids. Add banana and berries, rich in antioxidants, vitamins, and minerals.

Prep time: *About 20 minutes*

Yield: *2 servings*

1 to 2 tablespoons chia seeds

12 ounces water

1 banana, cut into 1-inch pieces

½ cup berries, any types

1 Grind chia seeds finely in a coffee grinder. Or use a hand grinder or put the seeds in a sealable plastic bag and break up with a rolling pin. Or use whole chia seeds.

2 In a blender, combine seeds and water. Blend 4 to 10 seconds on low speed.

3 Add banana pieces and berries to the blender. Blend on medium to high speed until smooth.

Tip: *Use frozen fruit for a thicker smoothie.*

Per serving: Calories 86 (From Fat 12); Fat 1g (Saturated 1g); Cholesterol 0mg; Sodium 2mg; Carbohydrate 19g (Dietary Fiber 4g); Protein 2g.

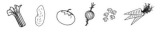

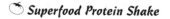

⟲ *Superfood Protein Shake*

This protein shake contains more than 25 grams of protein and three superfoods, making it a great snack at any time of the day. With the added chia, it will surely fill you up!

Prep time: *5 minutes*

Yield: *1 serving*

8 almonds, chopped

1 scoop of your favorite berry- or vanilla-flavored protein shake mix (look for mixes with fewer than 5g carbs and near 25g protein per serving)

8 to 10 ounces regular, light, or low-carb vanilla soy milk

1 tablespoon whole or ground chia seed

¼ cup frozen or fresh blueberries

Add the chopped almonds to blender and pulse a few times. Add the rest of the ingredients to the blender, and blend on low until smooth.

Per serving: *Calories 266 (From Fat 87); Fat 10g (Saturated 2g); Cholesterol 0mg; Sodium 394mg; Carbohydrate 13g (Dietary Fiber 7g); Protein 34g.*

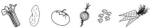

⟲ *Hummus and Pita*

Hummus is a spread made from garbanzo beans and sesame seed paste called tahini. Hummus is traditionally served with pita bread. It makes a delicious appetizer that's high in protein, fiber, and minerals.

Prep time: *About 10 minutes*

Yield: *8 servings*

6 cloves garlic

15-ounce can garbanzo
beans, rinsed and drained

3 tablespoons lemon juice

2 tablespoons olive oil

1½ tablespoons tahini

½ teaspoon salt

8 whole-wheat pitas, cut into
6 wedges

Process the garlic cloves in a food processer for 2 to
3 seconds. Add the remaining ingredients and process for 5 minutes, until smooth. Serve as a dip for
pita wedges.

Per serving: *Calories 210 (From Fat 59); Fat 7g (Saturated 1g);
Cholesterol 0mg; Sodium 509mg; Carbohydrate 33g (Dietary Fiber 5g);
Protein 7g.*

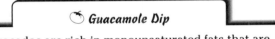

☜ *Guacamole Dip*

Avocados are rich in monounsaturated fats that are
good for your heart. Make this delicious dish extra-
healthy by choosing omega-3 enriched mayonnaise.

Prep time: *10 to 15 minutes*

Refrigeration time: *30 minutes*

Yield: *4 servings*

2 avocados, peeled and pitted

1 teaspoon salt

1 tablespoon lemon or lime
juice

1 teaspoon grated onion

½ teaspoon chili powder

½ cup light mayonnaise

1 In a large bowl, mash avocado with a fork.

2 Stir in salt, lemon or lime juice, onion, and chili
powder, and then mix in the mayonnaise. Cover and
refrigerate for 30 minutes before serving.

Per serving: *Calories 260 (From Fat 202); Fat 22g (Saturated 4g);
Cholesterol 11mg; Sodium 824mg; Carbohydrate 11g (Dietary Fiber
8g); Protein 3g.*

☃ Almond Brittle

This snack is made with plenty of almonds, which are an excellent source of vitamin E, magnesium, trypto-phan (an amino acid), and fats that help keep your heart healthy. This recipe is sugar-free (diabetes-friendly) and easy to prepare — a great idea for the holiday season. Double the recipe for bigger parties.

Prep time: *10 to 15 minutes*

Cooking time: *25 minutes*

Yield: *4 servings*

Nonstick cooking spray	1 tablespoon cinnamon
1 egg white	¼ cup sugar-free pancake syrup
¼ teaspoon salt	2 cups roasted almonds

1 Preheat oven to 350 degrees Fahrenheit. Line a baking sheet with foil, and spray the foil with nonstick cooking spray.

2 In a medium-sized metal bowl, beat the egg white until foamy and slightly thickened. You get quicker results with a hand mixer as opposed to whisking by hand.

3 Add the salt, cinnamon, and syrup to the egg white, and mix well.

4 Stir in the almonds, and then spread the mixture on the baking sheet.

5 Bake for 25 minutes until dry. Break into pieces, and store in an airtight container.

Per serving: *Calories 435 (From Fat 329); Fat 37g (Saturated 3g); Cholesterol 0mg; Sodium 210mg; Carbohydrate 18g (Dietary Fiber 9g); Protein 16g.*

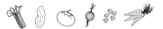

Starting off with superfood appetizers

An *appetizer* is a small amount of food or drink served before a meal to stimulate appetite. Sometimes they're so large and filling that instead of stimulating your appetite they satisfy it altogether. Keep portion control in mind when you make these.

Salmon Cakes

You can serve this great starter with confidence. Even people who aren't big fish eaters usually enjoy canned salmon. It's a great source of omega-3 fatty acids and protein. Oatmeal adds fiber, and parsley is a terrific source of vitamin C.

Prep time: About 20 minutes
Cooking time: 8 minutes
Yield: 5 servings

⅓ cup nonfat milk

2 egg whites

15-ounce can salmon, drained

1 cup whole-wheat bread crumbs

¾ cup quick-cooking oats (not instant or old-fashioned oats)

2 tablespoons chopped green onions

1 tablespoon chopped fresh dill

1 tablespoon chopped fresh parsley

¼ teaspoon paprika

¼ teaspoon salt

1 tablespoon olive oil

1 In a small bowl, beat together the milk and egg whites.

2 In a large bowl, combine the salmon, bread crumbs, oats, onions, dill, parsley, paprika, and salt, and mix well. Stir in the egg and milk mixture, and let it all stand for 5 minutes.

3 Shape the salmon mixture into 5 equally sized cakes, each about 1-inch thick.

4 Place a large skillet over medium heat, and add the olive oil. Sauté the salmon cakes until golden, about 4 minutes on each side.

Per serving: Calories 173 (From Fat 88); Fat 10g (Saturated 2g); Cholesterol 54mg; Sodium 542mg; Carbohydrate 4g (Dietary Fiber 1g); Protein 19g.

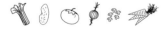

◌ *Spinach & Artichoke Pizza*

Pizza has never been healthier! This version contains garlic, flax, and spinach, so it has lots of vitamins, minerals, and healthy fats. Enjoy the rich flavor of the garlic, basil, and peppers.

Prep time: *20 minutes*

Cooking time: *5 to 8 minutes*

Yield: *4 to 6 servings*

1 tablespoon flax seed	*1 large portabella mushroom, thinly sliced*
2 cloves garlic, diced or pressed	
3 tablespoons olive oil, divided	*10 ounces fresh spinach leaves*
4 low-carb or whole-wheat wraps or tortillas	*1 teaspoon fresh basil leaves*
	14-ounce can artichoke hearts, drained and chopped
1 medium red bell pepper, seeded and cut into ¼-inch strips	*1½ cups shredded part-skim mozzarella cheese*

1 Preheat oven to 400 degrees Fahrenheit.

2 Grind the flax seed in a coffee grinder or small food processor. Combine it with the garlic and 1 tablespoon olive oil in a small bowl, and mix well.

3 Spread 1 teaspoon of the garlic mixture over each of the wraps.

4 In a medium skillet over medium heat, sauté the red pepper strips and mushrooms in the remaining olive oil for 5 minutes, until soft. Add the spinach leaves and sauté for another 2 minutes.

5 Layer the pepper and spinach mixture with the basil leaves and artichokes over the garlic mixture on each wrap, and top with cheese.

6 Bake for 5 to 8 minutes until golden brown and the cheese is melted. Cut into small wedges before serving.

Per serving: Calories 379 (From Fat 187); Fat 21g (Saturated 6g); Cholesterol 23mg; Sodium 577mg; Carbohydrate 26g (Dietary Fiber 11g); Protein 23g.

Salmon Lettuce Wraps

Salmon is rich in omega-3 fats and protein. This recipe could easily be a main dish, but when sliced into finger food it makes a great starter. It also contains tomatoes, garlic, and other fine herbs. Have leftovers as a snack the next day.

Prep time: *20 minutes*
Cooking time: *20 minutes*
Yield: *4 servings*

2 tablespoons fresh ginger, roughly chopped

¼ cup fresh cilantro

1 jalapeño pepper, seeded and roughly chopped

1 small onion, roughly chopped

2 cloves garlic, roughly chopped

2 tablespoons olive oil, divided

3 tablespoons fresh-squeezed lime juice

1 large tomato, roughly chopped

2 fresh salmon fillets (about 6 ounces each)

1 head iceberg or Bibb lettuce, or large spinach leaves

Lime wedges, for serving

1 Preheat broiler to high.

2 Combine the ginger, cilantro, jalapeño pepper, onion, garlic, 1 tablespoon olive oil, and lime juice in a food processor, and process until chopped and mixed. Add the tomato and process again. Transfer to a bowl, cover, and refrigerate.

3 Lightly coat salmon fillets with the rest of the olive oil, salt, and pepper. Place fillets on a foil-lined baking sheet and broil for 20 minutes, or until salmon is firm and pink.

4 Separate lettuce leaves from the head. Fill with small pieces of the flaked broiled salmon and the ginger mixture from Step 2. Top with fresh lime juice when serving.

Per serving: *Calories 140 (From Fat 53); Fat 6g (Saturated 1g); Cholesterol 32mg; Sodium 50mg; Carbohydrate 9g (Dietary Fiber 2g); Protein 14g.*

☙ Baked Spinach and Artichoke Dip

With the garlic and artichokes this becomes an appetizer of choice. You can serve it with low-carb wraps for dipping (bake for a few minutes until crispy) or substitute other superfoods as dippers, such as broccoli spears and celery.

Prep time: *20 minutes*
Cooking time: *20 minutes*
Yield: *4 servings*

Nonstick cooking spray	½ cup mayonnaise
1 pound frozen chopped spinach, thawed and drained	½ cup sour cream
2 tablespoons olive oil	2 cups part-skim shredded mozzarella cheese
1 clove garlic, minced	2 cups crumbled feta cheese
15-ounce can artichoke hearts, drained and chopped	2 tablespoons ground pepper
1 tablespoon red pepper flakes	

1 Preheat oven to 350 degrees. Spray a 1-quart casserole or baking dish with nonstick cooking spray and set aside.

2 In a large skillet over medium-high heat, sauté the spinach, olive oil, and garlic for 5 minutes.

3 Add to the skillet the remaining ingredients except for red pepper flakes, and mix well. Transfer the mixture to the casserole or baking dish, and bake for 20 to 25 minutes.

4 Sprinkle with red pepper flakes before serving.

Per serving: *Calories 699 (From Fat 510); Fat 57g (Saturated 21g); Cholesterol 100mg; Sodium 1,503mg; Carbohydrate 20g (Dietary Fiber 6g); Protein 31g.*

Delving into not-too-decadent desserts

It's what you've been waiting for — desserts! If you think any dessert with superfoods must be super taste-less, think again. Anytime you can get superfoods into your eating structure, you should do it. Read on for some super desserts you can serve with a smile.

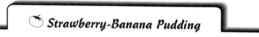

ᴄ *Strawberry-Banana Pudding*

This quick dessert is low in calories and carbohydrates, yet rich in antioxidants, vitamins, and minerals thanks to the almonds and strawberries. And it's easy to make!

Prep time: *10 minutes*

Yield: *1 serving*

3½-ounce container banana-flavored pudding (Snack Pack size)

4 strawberries, finely diced

1 tablespoon whipped topping

1 tablespoon finely crushed almonds

Stir together the pudding, strawberries, and whipped topping. Top with almonds.

Tip: *Feel free to use vanilla pudding also. If you are watching your weight, try "no sugar added" pudding.*

Per serving: *Calories 199 (From Fat 78); Fat 9g (Saturated 3g); Cholesterol 0mg; Sodium 150mg; Carbohydrate 29g (Dietary Fiber 3g); Protein 3g.*

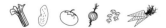

🐚 *Almond Puffs*

This is another great almond delight that's a delicious way to enjoy a superfood. Plus, it's diabetes-friendly! Although this recipe may not be as easy as the almond brittle, it's worth it. Plus, your kids will love them!

Prep time: *20 minutes*

Cooking time: *20 to 30 minutes*

Yield: *4 to 6 servings*

Nonstick cooking spray	*1 tablespoon vanilla extract*
4 egg whites	*½ teaspoon almond extract*
⅛ teaspoon salt	*½ cup toasted almonds, ground in food processor*
1½ cups sucralose sugar substitute	

1 Preheat oven to 250 degrees Fahrenheit. Spray 2 baking sheets with nonstick cooking spray.

2 Beat the egg whites with an electric mixer for a few minutes until they're creamy white and smooth. Add salt. Continue beating while slowly adding sugar substitute and extracts. Beat until the egg whites form stiff peaks (the points of beaten egg white should stand up on their own).

3 Fold in chopped almonds.

4 Use a teaspoon to drop batter onto cookie sheets, lifting the spoon at the end to create peaks.

5 Bake for 20 to 30 minutes until lightly brown and firm to the touch. Transfer to a wire rack to cool. Store in an airtight container.

Per serving: *Calories 129 (From Fat 54); Fat 6g (Saturated 1g); Cholesterol 0mg; Sodium 128mg; Carbohydrate 12g (Dietary Fiber 1g); Protein 6g.*

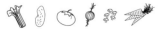

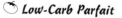 Low-Carb Parfait

This is a quick and tasty snack for low-carb dieters and, of course, diabetics. It contains chia and bananas and is so good it will satisfy even the toughest critic's sweet tooth.

Prep time: *10 minutes*

Yield: *1 serving*

3½-ounce container pudding in your favorite flavor, low sugar if possible	*3½-ounce container low-carb yogurt in your favorite flavor*
1 tablespoon whole chia seeds (you can grind them if you prefer)	*1 banana, cut into bite-sized pieces*
	1 tablespoon sugar-free whipped topping

1 In a small bowl, mix together the pudding and chia.

2 Layer yogurt and pudding in a dessert glass and top with banana and whipped topping.

Per serving: *Calories 354 (From Fat 48); Fat 5g (Saturated 3g); Cholesterol 10mg; Sodium 828mg; Carbohydrate 61g (Dietary Fiber 6g); Protein 15g.*

Chapter 7

Superfood Main Dishes, Salads, and Sides

. . . .

In This Chapter

▶ Planning main dishes: Good food and good conversation

▶ Making great superfood salads

▶ Preparing delicious and healthy side dishes

. . . .

*W*hen you're on the go, tracking what everyone is eating and whether you're getting the right balance of foods during the day can be hard. That's why it's important to plan and prepare healthy superfoods dinners for your family. Family dinners are a great opportunity to get everyone to eat healthily and gain back ground from the poor eating habits that both children and adults may indulge in during the day. And the same logic goes for the accompanying salads and side dishes you serve at dinner.

You can get superfoods in everything from salmon to pizza. After you get some creative meal ideas, you'll see how fun and easy it is to make healthy (and delicious) main dishes. In this chapter, we offer some easy recipes that cover a variety of superfoods — and will surely keep your family coming back for more!

Making the Most of Family Mealtime

Turn off the TV, let the phone go to voice mail, and disconnect from the Web, because it's time to sit down for an hour devoted to food and companionship. It just happens that dinner is the most consistent time for family gathering — the perfect time to get in touch with your family and find out what's going on in everyone's day. Getting everyone together for dinner may be a challenge, but try it every chance you get.

Several studies have looked at the importance of family mealtimes, for both children and adults. A study in the *Journal of the American Dietetic Association* showed that both children and parents strongly value family meals. Columbia University researchers found that children who ate more than five meals per week with their families had higher grades. Other studies have looked into school and work performance, drug use, and language skills, and have found similar positive outcomes associated with families who share several meals a week. A study published in the *Archives of Pediatric and Adolescent Medicine* claims that eating family meals may reduce the number of teens afflicted with eating disorders. Wow — all this from spending some quality family time around the table enjoying good food.

Obviously, dinner is a time to feed your bodies and your relationships. People who eat alone tend to eat less and may therefore suffer from malnutrition — an important fact to remember if you have friends and family members who spend most of their mealtimes alone. Invite them to join you when you can.

If you have trouble getting your family to the dinner table without simultaneously watching TV or attempting to scarf down the food and scram, you may have to get creative to get them into main meal festivities.

One way to keep the attendance up is to get the family involved in meal planning and preparation. Young children often love to cook, and they'll jump at the chance to help in the kitchen.

 Putting together a meal is a great accomplishment, especially when you're new to the kitchen, so be sure to compliment the chef.

Making a Statement with the Main Dish

The recipes for the main dishes in this chapter have a nice mix of superfoods that are sure to tantalize your taste buds! These recipes are easy to follow and a perfect way to get friends and family involved in the planning, cooking, and, most important, eating of healthy meals. You also find easy tricks for adding and substituting ingredients to get more nutritious superfoods into the recipes.

Too many are set on the idea that food that tastes good usually isn't good for you. Dinner is a perfect time to direct everyone's attention to the fun aspects of putting together a healthy meal. Let everyone know they're eating superfoods. Tell your family how the foods and ingredients contribute to good health. With these delicious superfoods meals, both young and old can discover that healthy eating can also taste good.

 When you cook for friends, offer them recipes for the dishes you prepare. Friends often want the recipe, but may be afraid to ask. Make it easy for them, and they can leave with a full belly and a fresh new superfoods dish for their own repertoire!

In this section, we have a few fish recipes that are always a great choice for tasty main dishes. However, we also include a nice mix of other meal options, whether you want a zesty burger, stir-fry, or a hot bowl of super stew.

Baked Salmon Fillets

Salmon is packed with the most omega-3 fatty acids. Even people who don't like fish are likely to enjoy salmon when you prepare it this way. Salmon is also low in saturated fat and a great source of protein, and it has a lot of B vitamins and magnesium.

Prep time: *About 15 minutes*

Cooking time: *Approximately 20 minutes*

Yield: *4 servings*

4 salmon fillets, 4 ounces each	*1 white onion, finely chopped*
3 tablespoons olive oil, divided	*2 tablespoons chopped fresh dill*
Salt and pepper	*1 teaspoon fresh lemon juice*

1 Preheat oven to 425 degrees Fahrenheit.

2 Rinse the salmon fillets under water and pat dry. Brush salmon fillets with 1 tablespoon olive oil, and sprinkle with salt and pepper.

3 Place fillets in baking dish. Bake for about 15 to 20 minutes, or until salmon is firm and flakes easily with a fork or knife.

4 Remove the salmon from the oven and cover to keep warm.

5 Heat a sauté pan to medium high, and add the remaining olive oil, onion, and fresh dill. Cook until the onions are soft and translucent.

6 Stir in fresh lemon juice.

7 Spoon sautéed sauce over salmon and serve.

Per serving: Calories 257 (From Fat 130); Fat 15g (Saturated 2g); Cholesterol 65mg; Sodium 230mg; Carbohydrate 6g (Dietary Fiber 1g); Protein 25g.

Baked Salmon with Sour Cream

The addition of garlic and onion give a great, savory taste to this fresh fish. You get healthy fats from the salmon and antioxidants and immune-boosting power from another superfood, garlic.

Prep time: *About 15 minutes*

Cooking time: *Approximately 20 minutes*

Yield: *4 servings*

4 salmon fillets, about 4 ounces each	*2 teaspoons finely chopped onion*
1 tablespoon olive oil	*1 clove garlic, minced*
Salt and pepper	*1 cup low-fat sour cream*
2 tablespoons fresh lemon juice	*1 bunch of parsley*

1 Preheat oven to 425 degrees Fahrenheit.

2 Rinse the salmon fillets under water and pat dry, and then place the salmon fillets in a baking dish. Lightly brush with olive oil, season with salt and pepper, and then sprinkle with lemon juice.

3 In a separate bowl, mix the onion and garlic together.

4 Spread sour cream on the fillets, and then the onion and garlic over the sour cream. Bake 15 to 20 minutes until firm, or until the salmon flakes easily with a knife or fork.

5 Garnish with parsley and serve.

Per serving: *Calories 395 (From Fat 161); Fat 18g (Saturated 6g); Cholesterol 117mg; Sodium 358mg; Carbohydrate 14g (Dietary Fiber 1g); Protein 42g.*

Black Bean Cilantro Lime Salmon

The last of our superfood salmon recipes offers another option for preparing a healthy salmon dish. Adding black beans increases the fiber content and adds to the already healthy benefits of the salmon.

Prep time: *About 15 minutes*

Cooking time: *Approximately 20 minutes*

Yield: *4 servings*

4 salmon fillets, about 4 ounces each	*½ cup black beans (canned beans are a suitable substitute, but we prefer fresh beans)*
2 tablespoons olive oil, divided	
Salt and pepper to taste	*1 to 2 tablespoons chopped fresh cilantro*
1 lime	
1 lemon	*1 to 2 tablespoons chopped fresh basil*
1 onion, chopped	

1 Preheat oven to 425 degrees Fahrenheit.

2 Place salmon fillets in a baking dish. Brush fillets with 1 tablespoon olive oil and season with salt and pepper.

3 Cut lime and lemon into wedges for squeezing.

4 Bake for 10 to 15 minutes, or until the salmon flakes when tested with a fork.

5 While salmon is baking, add remaining tablespoon olive oil, chopped onion, and black beans to small sauté pan. Sprinkle with salt and pepper to taste. Sauté on medium heat for 5 to 7 minutes until onions soften and beans are soft.

6 Top salmon fillets with beans and onion mixture, and squeeze fresh lime and lemon wedges over top.

7 Finish with chopped cilantro and basil, and serve.

Per serving: *Calories 375 (From Fat 122); Fat 14g (Saturated 2g); Cholesterol 97mg; Sodium 273mg; Carbohydrate 19g (Dietary Fiber 6g); Protein 43g.*

Trout Amandine

Trout has a mild flavor and is rich in omega-3 fatty acids; almonds are rich in healthy fats. Our version of trout amandine calls for poaching, which is a very healthful way to prepare fish.

Prep time: *About 10 minutes*

Cooking time: *17 to 19 minutes*

Yield: *2 servings*

¼ cup slivered almonds

½ cup dry white wine

⅓ cup lemon juice (or 2 to 3 fresh lemons, squeezed)

¼ cup chopped fresh parsley

¼ cup chopped green onions

¼ teaspoon salt

⅛ teaspoon pepper

2 fillets of trout (6 to 8 ounces each)

1 fresh lemon

1 Place almonds in small, nonstick skillet and toast over medium heat. Stir frequently until they're slightly brown, about 3 to 5 minutes. Remove from heat.

2 Pour wine, lemon juice, parsley, green onions, salt, and pepper into a large, nonstick skillet over medium heat and cook until the mixture begins to boil, about 4 minutes.

3 Reduce to low heat and add trout fillets. Cover the skillet to poach the fish until the flesh is opaque and flaky, about 10 minutes.

4 While fish is poaching, slice lemon.

5 Top trout fillets with almonds and a little poaching liquid, and serve with lemon slices.

Per serving: *Calories 298 (From Fat 131); Fat 15g (Saturated 2g); Cholesterol 97mg; Sodium 237mg; Carbohydrate 4g (Dietary Fiber 1g); Protein 37g.*

Basil Pesto and Broccoli Pasta with Chicken

Our pesto contains walnuts, which are a superfood, along with olive oil and garlic. Make it even more healthful by using whole-grain pasta.

Basil Pesto

Prep time: *About 10 minutes*

Yield: *1½ cups*

3 tablespoons walnuts

1½ tablespoons pine nuts

4 garlic cloves

3 cups fresh basil leaves, packed

¾ cup extra-virgin olive oil

⅓ cup grated Parmesan cheese

1 Place the walnuts, pine nuts, and garlic in a food processor. Process for 15 seconds.

2 Add the basil leaves, olive oil, and Parmesan cheese. Process again until the pesto is thoroughly puréed, about 10 seconds. Use or refrigerate in an airtight container for up to a week.

Per serving: *Calories 307 (From Fat 290); Fat 32g (Saturated 5g); Cholesterol 4mg; Sodium 95mg; Carbohydrate 3g (Dietary Fiber 1g); Protein 4g.*

Broccoli Pasta with Chicken

Prep time: *About 15 minutes*

Cooking time: *20 to 25 minutes*

Yield: *6 servings*

12 ounces dry penne or rigatoni pasta

3 tablespoons olive oil, divided

1 pound skinless, boneless chicken breast, cut into bite-sized pieces

1 red bell pepper, cut into bite-sized pieces

4 cups broccoli florets

1 tablespoon minced garlic

1 cup chopped tomatoes

¾ cup prepared basil pesto (see preceding recipe to make your own)

⅓ cup freshly grated Parmesan cheese

Salt and pepper to taste

1 Cook the pasta in a large pot of water for 8 to 10 minutes until tender but firm.

2 While pasta cooks, heat 2 tablespoons olive oil in a large, nonstick skillet over medium heat. Add chicken and red pepper, and cook for 5 to 10 minutes, or until chicken is cooked through. Remove from heat and transfer the chicken and pepper mixture to a large serving bowl.

3 Fill medium saucepan with water and bring to boil over medium-high heat. Blanch broccoli florets for 3 minutes, and then drain.

4 Pour remaining tablespoon of olive oil in the skillet used for the chicken and peppers. Add garlic, tomatoes, and pesto, and sauté for 2 minutes.

5 Add the pasta, broccoli, pesto mixture, and Parmesan cheese to the chicken and peppers. Toss to combine and add salt and pepper to taste.

Per serving: *Calories 544 (From Fat 233); Fat 26g (Saturated 5g); Cholesterol 47mg; Sodium 290mg; Carbohydrate 51g (Dietary Fiber 6g); Protein 30g.*

Tuna Melt Wraps

This sandwich recipe contains five superfoods: tuna, spinach, tomato, olive oil, and avocado. These warm wraps are easy to make and go nicely with a side salad or cup of soup. If you don't want to use a broiler, you can use a microwave.

Prep time: *About 10 minutes*

Cooking time: *2 to 3 minutes*

Yield: *2 servings*

2 whole-wheat tortillas	*½ cup diced tomato*
5 ounces canned tuna (regular or albacore), drained	*¼ cup diced avocado*
	2 teaspoons extra-virgin olive oil
½ cup shredded part-skim mozzarella cheese	*1 teaspoon balsamic vinegar*
1 cup fresh spinach leaves	*Salt and pepper to taste*

1 Preheat broiler to high.

2 Place tortillas on a baking sheet. Place half the tuna in the middle of each tortilla and sprinkle with cheese (dividing it between the two tortillas).

3 Place in the broiler until cheese is melted and tuna is warm, about 2 to 3 minutes. Remove from the broiler.

4 Transfer the tortillas to a clean cutting board. Add half of the spinach leaves, tomato, and avocado to each. Drizzle about 1 teaspoon of olive oil and balsamic vinegar over each. Add salt and pepper.

5 Fold up one quarter of each tortilla to form the bottom. Roll the sides in to form a cone shape, with the top open.

Tip: *You can make these melts in the microwave instead of the broiler if you prefer. To do so, place a tortilla on a microwave-safe plate and top with tuna and cheese. Cook on high until cheese is melted, about 1 to 1½ minutes (microwave oven times can vary greatly).*

Per serving: *Calories 312 (From Fat 118); Fat 13g (Saturated 4g); Cholesterol 38mg; Sodium 852mg; Carbohydrate 25g (Dietary Fiber 4g); Protein 29g.*

Tomato and Lentil Stew

Canned tomatoes are an excellent source of lycopene, which is good for your heart and prostate. Lentils are rich in fiber, folate, and protein. This superfood stew can be served as a meal with a small side salad and a slice of hearty, whole-grain bread.

Prep time: About 20 minutes

Cooking time: 40 minutes

Yield: 4 servings

1 tablespoon olive oil	½ teaspoon crushed red pepper
1 medium onion, finely chopped	½ cup dry red wine
4 medium carrots, diced	15-ounce can chopped tomatoes
4 medium celery ribs, diced	¾ cup dry red lentils
2 to 3 garlic cloves, crushed	4 cups low-sodium chicken or vegetable broth
¾ teaspoon dried basil	
¾ teaspoon dried thyme	Salt and pepper to taste

1 Heat oil in a Dutch oven or large soup pot. Add onion, carrots, celery, and garlic, and cook over low heat for about 5 minutes until soft, stirring occasionally.

2 Stir in basil, thyme, red pepper, red wine, tomatoes, and lentils. Cook for another 5 minutes, stirring constantly.

3 Add broth and bring to a boil. Reduce to low heat and simmer gently for 25 to 30 minutes, or until lentils are soft. Add salt and pepper to taste.

Tip: For slightly thicker or creamier soup, stir the soup with a whisk for about 30 seconds to break up the lentils, thickening the soup.

Per serving: Calories 255 (From Fat 46); Fat 5g (Saturated 1g); Cholesterol 4mg; Sodium 491mg; Carbohydrate 40g (Dietary Fiber 11g); Protein 14g.

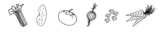

⟲ Southwestern Black Bean Burgers

Hamburgers are a family favorite; however, they're high in saturated fat, and that's not good for you. Our Southwestern Black Bean Burgers are rich in antioxidants, vitamins, and fiber, and low in calories. These burgers can also be cooked ahead of time and reheated when you're ready to eat.

Prep time: *About 10 minutes*

Cooking time: *10 minutes*

Yield: *4 servings*

15- to 16-ounce can black beans, rinsed and drained	1 teaspoon ground cumin
⅓ cup chopped red onion	½ teaspoon hot pepper sauce (such as Tabasco)
¼ cup chopped fresh cilantro	Salt and pepper to taste
¼ cup dry, whole-wheat bread crumbs	Canola oil or nonstick cooking spray
2 tablespoons chunky salsa or green chili sauce	4 whole-wheat hamburger buns

1 In a large bowl, mash the beans. Stir in the onion, cilantro, bread crumbs, salsa, cumin, and hot pepper sauce. Add salt and pepper.

2 Moisten your hands with water. Shape the bean mixture into four 3-inch burgers.

3 Oil or spray a large, nonstick skillet and place over medium heat. When skillet is hot, add the burgers and cook until lightly browned on the bottom, about 5 minutes. Turn and cook for 5 minutes longer, or until heated through.

4 Serve on whole-wheat hamburger buns.

Tip: *If you can't find ready-made whole-wheat bread crumbs, you can easily make them with 1 slice of whole-wheat bread in a food processor.*

Per serving: *Calories 199 (From Fat 23); Fat 3g (Saturated 0g); Cholesterol 0mg; Sodium 617mg; Carbohydrate 38g (Dietary Fiber 9g); Protein 9g.*

Chicken or Beef Fajitas with Avocado Sauce

This is a great recipe if you're hosting a party and aren't sure whether the guests would prefer beef or chicken. The key is the superfood avocado sauce that goes great with either one. This sauce combines garlic and avocado — two great superfoods.

Prep time: About 20 minutes

Cooking time: 10 to 15 minutes

Yield: 6 servings

Six to eight 8-inch or larger whole-grain tortillas

1 tablespoon olive oil

2 yellow or red bell peppers, cut into thin strips

1 medium onion, thinly sliced

2 tablespoons fajita seasoning

¼ cup water

4 boneless, skinless chicken breasts cut into thin strips, or 1 to 2 pounds of flank steak or other steak of choice sliced into thin strips, or half beef and half chicken

2 medium avocados, peeled, seeded, and sliced

½ medium onion, chopped

2 tablespoons lemon juice

1 clove garlic, minced

¼ teaspoon dried cilantro or 1 tablespoon chopped fresh cilantro

½ teaspoon salt

¼ teaspoon pepper

Shredded cheese and lettuce (optional)

1 Preheat oven to 425 degrees Fahrenheit.

2 Wrap the stack of tortillas in foil and place them in oven for 10 to 15 minutes.

3 Heat a large, nonstick skillet on high; add olive oil, peppers, and sliced onion, and sauté until vegetables begin to soften, about 3 minutes.

4 Mix fajita seasoning and water in a small bowl, and then pour the mixture into the skillet. Add the meat and sautéed vegetables, and cook for about 5 to 10 minutes until the meat is cooked through.

5 Make the avocado sauce by placing avocados, chopped onion, lemon juice, garlic, cilantro, salt, and pepper into a food processor; cover and blend until well mixed.

6 Serve the meat and vegetables on individual tortillas, and spoon avocado sauce on top. Top with shredded cheese and lettuce as desired.

Per serving: *Calories 338 (From Fat 133); Fat 15g (Saturated 3g); Cholesterol 49mg; Sodium 373mg; Carbohydrate 33g (Dietary Fiber 8g); Protein 23g.*

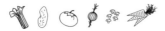

Turkey Chili

This recipe features the superfoods tomatoes, kidney beans, and garlic. The lean ground turkey keeps it low-fat and good for you.

Prep time: *About 15 minutes*

Cooking time: *40 to 55 minutes*

Yield: *8 servings*

1½ teaspoons olive oil	½ teaspoon salt
1 medium onion, chopped	½ teaspoon ground black pepper
1 pound lean ground turkey	16-ounce can kidney beans, rinsed and drained
2 tablespoons chili powder	
1 tablespoon chopped fresh cilantro	1 cup water
	1 cup beer
½ teaspoon paprika	28-ounce can crushed tomatoes
½ teaspoon dried oregano	4-ounce can green chiles, undrained
½ teaspoon ground cayenne pepper	1 tablespoon minced garlic

1 Heat the oil in a large soup pot over medium heat. Add the onion and cook for about 3 to 4 minutes.

2 Add the ground turkey to the onions, and then stir in the chili powder, cilantro, paprika, oregano, cayenne pepper, salt, and black pepper. Cook until the meat is evenly browned, about 5 minutes.

3 In a small bowl, mash approximately half of the beans.

4 Add the water and beer to the pot, and stir in the tomatoes, mashed and whole kidney beans, green chiles, and garlic. Stir until combined.

5 Reduce heat to low, cover, and simmer 30 to 45 minutes before serving. Stir occasionally.

Per serving: *Calories 158 (From Fat 16); Fat 2g (Saturated 0g); Cholesterol 37mg; Sodium 456mg; Carbohydrate 18g (Dietary Fiber 4g); Protein 18g.*

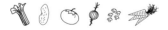

Pork Chops and Apples

Pork chops are a good source of selenium and B vitamins. This superfoods recipe adds the goodness of apples and pecans, plus raisins and honey for a touch of sweetness.

Prep time: *About 10 minutes*

Cooking time: *10 to 15 minutes*

Yield: *4 servings*

Nonstick cooking spray

Four 4-ounce boneless pork chops, ½ inch thick, trimmed of fat

½ cup finely chopped onion

1 large tart apple, such as Macintosh, Yellow Delicious, Rome, or Winesap, cored and finely chopped

¼ cup raisins

¼ cup chopped pecans

½ cup low-sodium chicken broth

½ cup apple juice

3 tablespoons honey

2 teaspoons Dijon mustard

¼ teaspoon dried thyme

¼ teaspoon cinnamon

1 tablespoon water

1 teaspoon cornstarch

1 Spray a large skillet with nonstick cooking spray and place over medium-high heat. Add the chops and cook until done, at least 4 to 5 minutes per side, or to an internal temperature of 180 degrees Fahrenheit. Transfer the pork chops to a plate and cover with foil to keep warm.

2 While the chops are cooking, spray a medium saucepan with nonstick cooking spray and place over medium-high heat. Add the onion to the pan and sauté 2 to 3 minutes, until it starts to soften, stirring continuously.

3 Add the apple slices to the onion and sauté until the apples are tender, about 3 to 5 minutes, stirring continuously.

4 Add the raisins and pecans to the onion and apple mixture. Stir in the broth, apple juice, honey, mustard, thyme, and cinnamon; cook for 5 minutes.

5 Mix water and cornstarch in a small bowl and add to the apple mixture. Stir until thickened and glossy, about 1 minute. Serve over chops.

Per serving: *Calories 349 (From Fat 116); Fat 13g (Saturated 3g); Cholesterol 67mg; Sodium 241mg; Carbohydrate 36g (Dietary Fiber 3g); Protein 25g.*

Tofu Stir-Fry

Tofu is made from soybeans and works well as a substitute for meat in stir-fry dishes. Our tofu stir-fry also contains olive oil, broccoli, and carrots, along with other healthful vegetables, which make it a delicious superfoods meal.

Prep time: *About 20 minutes*

Cooking time: *10 minutes*

Yield: *4 servings*

1 tablespoon olive oil

¼ cup cornstarch

16-ounce package extra firm tofu, drained and cut into cubes

½ medium onion, sliced

2 cloves garlic, finely chopped

1 tablespoon minced fresh ginger

2 cups broccoli florets

1 carrot, peeled and sliced

1 green bell pepper, seeded and cut into strips

1 small head bok choy, chopped

1 cup sliced fresh mushrooms

1 cup chopped canned bamboo shoots, drained

½ teaspoon crushed red pepper

½ cup water

¼ cup rice wine vinegar

2 tablespoons honey

2 tablespoons soy sauce

1 In a large skillet or wok, heat oil over medium-high heat. In a small bowl, toss tofu cubes in cornstarch to coat. Add tofu to skillet and sauté until golden brown, about 2 to 3 minutes, stirring occasionally.

2 Stir in onion, garlic, and ginger, and sauté for 1 minute.

3 Stir in broccoli, carrot, and bell pepper, and sauté for 2 minutes. Stir in bok choy, mushrooms, bamboo shoots, and crushed red pepper. Heat through, about 5 minutes, stirring continuously. Remove from heat.

4 In a small saucepan, combine water, rice wine vinegar, honey, and soy sauce, and bring to a simmer, stirring constantly. Pour over stir-fry mixture, toss, and serve.

Per serving: *Calories 235 (From Fat 103); Fat 11g (Saturated 2g); Cholesterol 0mg; Sodium 508mg; Carbohydrate 21g (Dietary Fiber 5g); Protein 18g.*

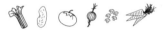

Filling Your Plate: Super Salad and Side Dish Recipes

Salads and sides dishes are perfect for introducing superfoods into your lifestyle. In this section, we offer some tips for making delicious and healthy salads and side dishes, along with some of our favorite recipes.

We suggest you eat five to nine servings of fruits and vegetables of different colors every day to get a variety of antioxidant-rich phytochemicals, fiber, and nutrients. You can get several of those servings by making salads and side dishes that include some of the fruit and vegetable superfoods.

The ingredients and cooking method called for in a recipe determine how healthy the resulting side or salad will be. When you page through your cookbooks (or surf online) to find healthy salads and side dishes, look for recipes that include

> ✔ Fruits, vegetables, or legumes as main ingredients

> ✔ Healthful oils such as olive, walnut, or canola oil

> ✔ Only small amounts of sugar (or, better yet, none at all)

> ✔ Cooking methods that don't add extra fat and calories — baking, roasting, sautéing, and stir-frying

 If your favorite recipes don't include superfoods as ingredients, you can make them a little bit healthier by making substitutions like these:

> ✔ Use dried cranberries instead of raisins in slaws and salads.

> ✔ Substitute albacore tuna for chicken in salads.

> ✔ Start your salad with raw spinach leaves instead of iceberg lettuce.

> ✔ Top your salad with pecans or sunflower seeds instead of croutons.

> ✔ Replace vegetable oil with olive oil.

These recipes are all created with superfoods, along with other ingredients that are good for you. Many of them don't require any cooking time — all you need are a few ingredients and a few minutes to prepare them. And several of them are easy enough that you can enlist the help of your children.

Serving up super salads

Serve up a healthy salad to go alongside a sandwich at lunch or in place of a vegetable at dinner. You can also enjoy one of these salads as a delicious and healthy afternoon snack — say, when you're hungry and dinner is still three hours away.

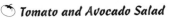 **Tomato and Avocado Salad**

Tomatoes, avocados, and olive oil offer a delicious combination of vitamins, antioxidants, and healthful oils — truly a heart-healthy dish!

Prep time: *About 5 to 15 minutes*

Yield: *4 servings*

1 avocado, peeled, pitted, and sliced	½ cup olive oil
2 small tomatoes, each cut into 8 wedges	2 tablespoons lime juice
1 small sweet onion, thinly sliced	2 tablespoons chopped fresh cilantro
	Salt and pepper to taste

1 Arrange avocado, tomatoes, and onion on a serving plate in alternating fashion.

2 Whisk together the olive oil, lime juice, and cilantro. Pour the dressing over the salad, and add salt and pepper to taste.

Vary It!: *If fresh cilantro isn't available or isn't to your liking, you can use parsley instead.*

Per serving: *Calories 322 (From Fat 301); Fat 33g (Saturated 5g); Cholesterol 0mg; Sodium 150mg; Carbohydrate 7g (Dietary Fiber 5g); Protein 2g.*

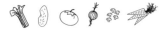

◌ *Refreshing Bean Salad*

This salad packs a lot of punch with antioxidant-rich vegetables. Red onions are a good source of quercetin, a powerful bioflavonoid antioxidant. The beans add plenty of protein and fiber to keep you feeling full without adding lots of calories.

Prep time: *About 15 minutes*

Refrigeration time: *At least 3 hours*

Yield: *4 servings*

1 red onion, peeled and chopped	*1 cup red kidney beans, rinsed and drained*
1 red bell pepper, chopped	*1 sprig parsley, chopped*
2 15-ounce cans cut green beans, drained	*½ fresh lemon, squeezed*
	3 tablespoons olive oil
15-ounce can soybeans, rinsed and drained	*½ cup balsamic vinegar*

1 Toss beans, onion, pepper, and parsley in a large bowl, mixing well.

2 In a small bowl, whisk together the lemon juice, vinegar, and olive oil. Poor over the bean mixture, and toss to combine. Cover and refrigerate for a minimum of 3 hours prior to serving.

Tip: *You can use rice vinegar instead of balsamic to preserve the coloring of the vegetables.*

Per serving: *Calories 271 (From Fat 129); Fat 14g (Saturated 2g); Cholesterol 0mg; Sodium 578mg; Carbohydrate 29g (Dietary Fiber 8g); Protein 11g.*

☙ *Cucumber and Tomato Salad*

Tomatoes shine as the superfood star of this recipe, and they're combined with two other superfoods: garlic and olive oil. The rest of the ingredients are good for you, too. Cucumbers add vitamin C and minerals, and feta cheese adds protein and calcium.

Prep time: *About 15 minutes*

Yield: *4 servings*

2 cucumbers, peeled and thinly sliced	½ teaspoon minced garlic
½ cup red onion, thinly sliced	⅓ cup red wine vinegar
2 large tomatoes, cut into small wedges or diced	2 tablespoons olive oil
¼ cup crumbled feta cheese	1 teaspoon chopped fresh oregano
	Salt and pepper to taste

1 In a large mixing bowl, combine the cucumber, onion, tomato, and feta cheese.

2 In a small bowl, whisk together the garlic, vinegar, oil, oregano, salt, and pepper. Add to the cucumber and tomato mixture, and toss to combine. Cover and refrigerate until you're ready to serve.

Per serving: *Calories 126 (From Fat 84); Fat 9g (Saturated 2g); Cholesterol 8mg; Sodium 263mg; Carbohydrate 9g (Dietary Fiber 2g); Protein 3g.*

Caribbean Bean Salad

Make any meal a super meal with this salad — it contains four of our superfoods. The nutrients and phytochemicals come from tomatoes, oranges, black beans, and soybeans. Romaine lettuce is rich in vitamins and minerals and super-low in calories.

Prep time: *About 15 minutes*

Yield: *4 servings*

4 cups chopped romaine
lettuce

1 medium red onion, diced

1 tomato, chopped

1 cucumber, peeled, seeded,
and sliced

1 orange, peeled and sliced

½ cup canned black beans,
rinsed and drained

½ cup canned soybeans,
rinsed and drained

1 tablespoon olive oil

3 tablespoons red wine
vinegar

1 teaspoon dried oregano

Black pepper to taste

1 In a large bowl, combine the lettuce, onion, tomato,
cucumber, orange, and beans.

2 In a small bowl, whisk together the olive oil, vinegar,
and oregano. Pour over the vegetable and bean mixture, and toss to combine. Add pepper to taste.

Per serving: *Calories 143 (From Fat 49); Fat 6g (Saturated 1g);
Cholesterol 0mg; Sodium 157mg; Carbohydrate 20g (Dietary Fiber 7g);
Protein 7g.*

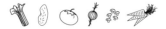

ᕙ *Strawberry and Spinach Salad*

Strawberries, spinach, and almonds give this salad a lot of nutrients, including vitamin C and calcium. Sesame seeds add trace minerals copper and manganese that help keep your bones healthy. The sweet taste of the strawberries in this recipe helps introduce kids to superfoods.

Prep time: *About 30 minutes*

Yield: *4 servings*

2 tablespoons sugar

½ cup olive oil

¼ cup balsamic vinegar

¼ teaspoon Worcestershire sauce

1 quart strawberries, hulled and sliced

10 ounces fresh spinach, rinsed and dried

¼ cup sliced almonds

3 tablespoons toasted sesame seeds

1 In a small bowl, whisk together sugar, olive oil, balsamic vinegar, and Worcestershire sauce.

2 In a large bowl, combine the strawberries, spinach, almonds, and sesame seeds. Just before serving, add the dressing to the salad, and toss to combine.

Per serving: *Calories 783 (From Fat 302); Fat 34g (Saturated 4g); Cholesterol 0mg; Sodium 125mg; Carbohydrate 124g (Dietary Fiber 9g); Protein 5g.*

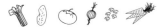

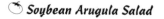

☙ Soybean Arugula Salad

This salad contains lots of nutrients, antioxidants, fiber, and healthy fats. Arugula is an aromatic salad green that's low in calories and high in vitamins A and C.

Prep time: *About 20 minutes, plus 2 to 3 hours for flavors to combine*

Cooking time: *5 minutes*

Yield: *4 servings*

Two 15-ounce cans of soybeans, undrained	*1 tablespoon red wine vinegar*
1 teaspoon salt, divided	*3 tablespoons sherry vinegar*
1 teaspoon ground black pepper, divided	*⅓ cup olive oil*
1 teaspoon garlic powder	*3 diced Roma tomatoes*
2 garlic cloves	*¼ cup chopped black olives*
¾ teaspoon dried rosemary	*1 large bunch (about 5 ounces) of arugula, stems removed, and chopped*
1 teaspoon dried oregano	*¼ cup grated parmesan cheese*

1 Heat the beans in medium saucepan over medium heat and add ½ teaspoon salt, ½ teaspoon black pepper, and garlic powder. Remove from the heat when the beans start to bubble. Strain the beans after cooking.

2 In a blender or small food processor, place garlic cloves, rosemary, oregano, vinegars, ½ teaspoon salt, and ½ teaspoon pepper. Blend while slowly adding olive oil until the mixture is emulsified.

3 In a large bowl, combine the beans, tomatoes, and olives. Pour dressing over it and toss to combine. Cover and let sit for 2 to 3 hours to let the flavors come together. Serve at room temperature.

4 Immediately before serving, mix in chopped arugula and add freshly grated parmesan.

Per serving: *Calories 318 (From Fat 206); Fat 23g (Saturated 3g); Cholesterol 4mg; Sodium 754mg; Carbohydrate 16g (Dietary Fiber 7g); Protein 13g.*

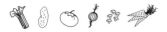

Creating super side dishes

These side dishes are loaded with nutrients and anti-oxidants. Serve them alongside grilled salmon or tuna steaks for super-duper healthy meals.

○ *Roasted Kale*

Kids love crispy foods, so this side dish is a good way to introduce picky eaters to green vegetables. Kale is a great source of vitamins A and C and has lots of calcium and iron. This recipe is so easy, even little kids can help.

Prep time: *About 10 minutes*

Cooking time: *15 to 20 minutes*

Yield: *2 servings*

1 bunch kale (about 1 pound)	2 cloves garlic, crushed
1 tablespoon olive oil	Sea salt and pepper to taste

1 Preheat oven to 375 degrees Fahrenheit. Rinse the kale in running water and shake to dry. Tear leaves into smaller pieces, and discard tough rib sections.

2 In a small bowl, whisk together the olive oil, garlic, salt, and pepper.

3 In a large bowl, toss the kale leaves with the olive oil mixture. Spread leaves on a baking sheet. Bake for 15 to 20 minutes, turning the kale every 7 to 8 minutes. It's done when the leaves are crispy and bright green with just a little brown around the edges.

Per serving: *Calories 132 (From Fat 70); Fat 8g (Saturated 1g); Cholesterol 0mg; Sodium 346mg; Carbohydrate 15g (Dietary Fiber 5g); Protein 5g.*

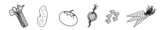

◌ *Orange Ginger Baby Carrots*

Carrots and oranges give this side dish a lot of vitamins and antioxidants. Ginger has been used as a digestive aid for centuries. This recipe is great for kids who are still learning to love vegetables, and it's so easy they can help. Teaching kids to cook is a great way to get them interested in trying new foods.

Prep time: *About 5 minutes*

Cooking time: *15 minutes*

Yield: *5 servings*

2 tablespoons canola oil	¾ cup orange juice
1 pound baby carrots	Salt and pepper to taste
2 teaspoons minced ginger (available already minced in jars)	

1 Heat oil in large skillet over medium heat. Add carrots, ginger, and orange juice, and bring to boil.

2 Reduce heat and simmer until carrots are tender, about 15 minutes. Add salt and pepper to taste.

Per serving: *Calories 108 (From Fat 49); Fat 6g (Saturated 1g); Cholesterol 0mg; Sodium 165mg; Carbohydrate 14g (Dietary Fiber 2g); Protein 1g.*

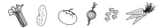

☞ Green Beans with Sun-Dried Tomatoes

Sun-dried tomatoes packed in olive oil contain lycopene, which is good for your heart (so is the olive oil). Green beans are low in calories and rich in vitamins and minerals. This side dish is easy to make, especially if you buy frozen green beans.

Prep time: *About 5 to 10 minutes*

Cooking time: *15 to 20 minutes*

Yield: *5 servings*

1 pound green beans, fresh or frozen

2 tablespoons olive oil

½ cup oil-packed sun-dried tomatoes, drained and minced

½ teaspoon oregano

2 tablespoons lemon juice

Salt and pepper to taste

1 Fill a pot with water and bring to a boil. Prepare green beans by boiling or steaming until tender-crisp, about 5 to 10 minutes. Drain and set aside.

2 Add olive oil and tomatoes to a large skillet over medium heat and stir until tomatoes are heated through, about 1 to 2 minutes. Stir in green beans and oregano, and cook for 1 to 2 minutes.

3 Transfer to a serving dish and sprinkle with lemon juice. Add salt and pepper to taste.

Per serving: *Calories 95 (From Fat 53); Fat 6g (Saturated 1g); Cholesterol 0mg; Sodium 232mg; Carbohydrate 11g (Dietary Fiber 4g); Protein 3g.*

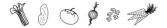

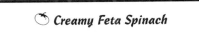

Creamy Feta Spinach

Dark green spinach is rich with calcium, vitamin K, folate, and antioxidants. This side dish also gives your family calcium and protein with the parmesan and feta cheese.

Prep time: *About 10 minutes*

Cooking time: *7 minutes*

Yield: *4 servings*

¾-ounce package of fresh dill, chopped

½ onion, minced

1 garlic clove, minced

1 tablespoon olive oil

7½-ounce can chopped spinach, drained; or 10-ounce box chopped frozen spinach, cooked

according to package instructions and drained

¼ cup grated parmesan cheese

¼ cup crumbled feta cheese

Freshly grated parmesan cheese (optional)

1 In a large saucepan over medium heat, sauté the dill, onion, and garlic in olive oil for 5 minutes.

2 Mix in the spinach, and then fold in both cheeses.

3 Serve topped with more parmesan cheese, if desired.

Per serving: *Calories 74 (From Fat 34); Fat 4g (Saturated 2g); Cholesterol 12mg; Sodium 251mg; Carbohydrate 6g (Dietary Fiber 3g); Protein 6g.*

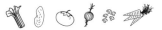

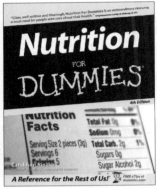
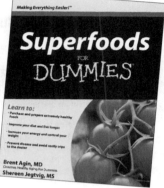
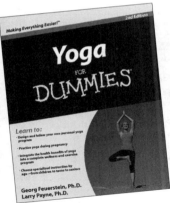
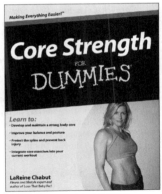

After you've read the Pocket Edition, look for the original Dummies book on the topic. The handy Contents at a Glance below highlights the information you'll get when you purchase a copy of *Superfoods For Dummies* — available wherever books are sold, or visit dummies.com.

Contents at a Glance